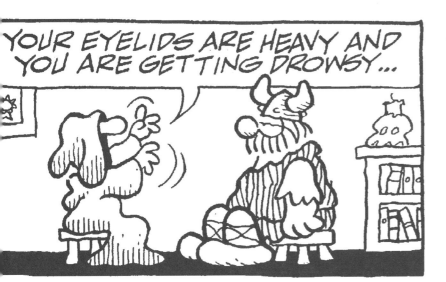

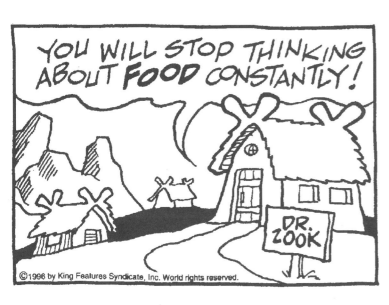

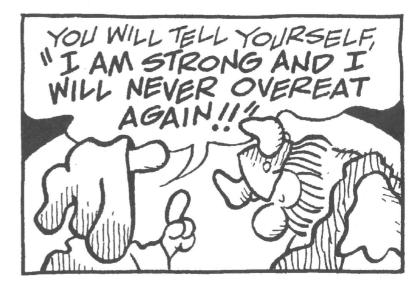

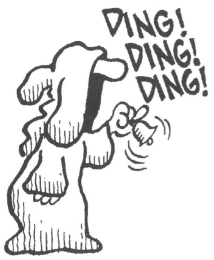

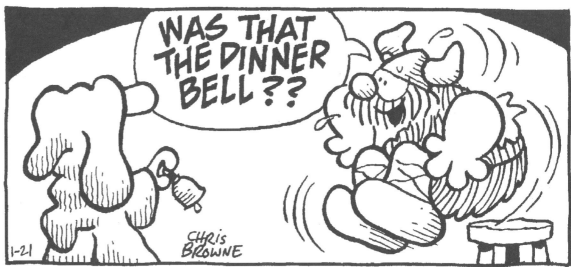

CHRIS BROWNE

1-21

FAT CHANCE
Your Best Chance for Permanent Weight Loss

Here's What People Are Saying About
FAT CHANCE:

"I can't put into words what I learned from Fat Chance!
Many thanks for steering my eighty-year-old bones in the right direction."
—Virginia Gerber

"What I like about this program is you can eat the foods you like,
making simple modifications, without losing the taste—unlike other weight
reduction programs. I would recommend it to anyone!"
—Dee Filippone

"Good to eat and good for you are no longer separate things at my table."
—Sherri Ilse

"Diet without feeling like you are on a diet.
Joan and Annette stress moderation not deprivation."
—Francesca Colombini

"Joan and Annette have combined their exceptional talent to
produce insightful and workable solutions for people with a desire
to eat good food and keep healthy."
—George W. Brown

"This straightforward, intelligent reality check on nutrition
and exercise is presented with so much enthusiasm, not only do you know you
can do it—you know you are going to enjoy it so much it will become a
permanent part of your lifestyle."
—Sandra McGaughey

FAT *Chance*

Your *Best* Chance for Permanent Weight Loss

JOAN CORTOPASSI • ANNETTE CAIN

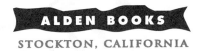

ALDEN BOOKS

STOCKTON, CALIFORNIA

Library of Congress Cataloging-in-Publication Data
Cortopassi, Joan, 1936–
      Fat Chance: your (best) chance for permanent weight loss / by Joan Cortopassi
and Annette Cain.
          p. cm.
      Includes recipe index.
      Includes bibliographical references.
      ISBN 0-9649496-0-1
      1. Weight loss. I. Cain, Annette, 1965- . II. Title.
RM222.2.C6445 1996   95-48221 CIP
613.2'5–dc20

Printed in the United States of America.

FIRST EDITION
1 2 3 4 5 6 7 8 9 10

DESIGN: JENNIFER WEBER
PRODUCTION: MELANIE HAAGE
EDITOR: COLIN INGRAM

To All of Our
Hard-Working Angels

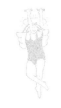

Acknowledgments

We would like to say a big THANKS to all of our wonderful students for giving us their feedback (no pun intended), for asking great questions and for sharing their ideas with us. Their enthusiasm and successful weight loss gave us the courage and the energy to continually try to improve our classes and to write this book to share the knowledge with others. Also, a special thanks to Colin Ingram, our copy editor, for burning the midnight oil and using his magic to help us create a fun and complete message. He kept us balanced and played the part of devil's advocate quite well. This book wouldn't be complete without also thanking the following people, without whose support we never could have completed such a daunting task as writing a book:

Alder Market
Ann Bell
Carmen Davis
Christy Morgan
Anne Hayes
Cullen Curtiss
Dick Darling
Don Lenz
Dr. Les Kadis
George and
Marilyn Brown
Georgia Hughes
Jennifer Weber
JoAnn Weir
John Cady
Julie Ambrose
Karen Behnke
Kent Lacin
Lana Rogerson
Lorene Freggiaro

Lauri Merrill, M.S., P.T. and
Monty Merrill, M.S., P.T., O.C.S.,
of Lodi Physical Therapy
Martha Mueller
Mary Bennett
Maxwell's Book Mark
Melanie Haage
Pat McCormick
Patty Kaul
Peggy Guttieri
San Tomo
Sandy Ervine
Saundra Kane
SFFFS
Sherri Smith and everyone at
Wine & Roses Country Inn
Stephanie Prima Serantopulos
of The Savory Thymes
Tony Ramirez of Ram Studio
Vicky Freggiaro

And, last but not least, to our favorite "angels," Dino Cortopassi
and Greg Rhines, for their eternal love and support!

CONTENTS

CONTENTS

CONTENTS

PART EIGHT

The Icing on the Cake

ix

PART NINE

Recipes (Yum!)

THY FOOD SHALL BE THE REMEDY.

—Hippocrates c. 460–377 B.C.

Meet the Cook and the Trainer

Joan Cortopassi, *The Cook*, was born and raised in Stockton, California and graduated from the University of the Pacific with a Bachelor of Science degree in Physical Education and Health. Living in the country and married to an Italian farmer and food processor, Joan has always enjoyed providing her guests with delicious, health-promoting meals. Joan's four children and eight grandchildren have taken up the family interest in fine food and now compete for space in the kitchen to help with the cooking.

As an active participant in the family business, Joan has had the responsibility and the fun of developing and testing new recipes for company products. For food shows, fund-raisers, business dinners and extended family dinners, she supervises the preparation of meals for several thousand people each year.

Joan is an active member of the San Francisco Professional Food Society, the American Institute of Wine and Food and the International Association of Culinary Professionals, as well as a Regent of the University of the Pacific. She is a lifelong devotee of tasty and healthy cooking, and teaching the art of delicious, low fat cooking is an enjoyable way for her to share her extensive knowledge.

Annette Cain, *The Trainer*, was born in San Francisco and graduated from the University of California at Davis with a Bachelor of Science degree in Nutrition Science. Annette's interest quickly expanded to include fitness, and she has worked for several years developing weight management and exercise programs. She is certified by the Aerobics and Fitness Association of America (AFAA) as a personal trainer, with an additional certification in weight room instruction.

1

Annette has always had a strong commitment to promoting wellness. She gives lectures and workshops on diet and fitness and is the nutrition editor of a local food journal. She is a volunteer health educator for the American Heart Association and is a member of the American College of Sports Medicine (ACSM) as well as several other professional groups.

In addition to her professional life, Annette runs in races from 5000 meters up to marathons and competes in triathlons. She is currently training for an "Ironman" distance triathlon (a 2.4-mile swim, a 112-mile bike ride, followed by a 26.2-mile run).

Low Fat Chat

Joan: I've always loved good food, but I was frustrated, year after year, with weight problems. I'm so used to preparing and eating really tasty food that I just didn't want to give it up. When I met Annette, in 1992, she helped me get going on a fat tracking and fitness program, and I ended up losing twenty pounds—permanently! I could hardly believe I'd finally found something that worked!

Annette: We were a perfect match. In addition to our common interest in low fat cooking, Joan brought her years of experience in making really delicious dishes. Her cooking techniques and her use of low fat food substitutions were very impressive. Joan can make anything taste great!

Joan: One of the things that helped me stay on my weight-loss program was Annette's approach to fitness. She made it a fun task, rather than an unpleasant chore. I actually looked forward to my daily exercise—and I still do now.

Annette: The more we worked together, the more we realized we had a formula for success. One of the ways we tested our techniques was by giving low fat cooking classes. In these classes, which are still ongoing, each participant gets to taste and evaluate our flavorful, low fat recipes. The response to our classes has been overwhelming, and the food is so tasty and easy to prepare that we have had more requests to attend than we can handle.

But this is only part of the combination needed for permanent weight loss. Last year we were able to develop a comprehensive program which demonstrated why restrictive diets don't work, and how the *right* combination of nutrition and exercise is necessary for weight loss to be permanent. We gradually put together a program that achieves permanent weight loss—no more ups and downs—

Joan: and no deprivation!

Annette: It's a program that really works. And it's enjoyable and comfortable.

Joan: What about "no pain, no gain?"

Annette: Out of date, unnecessary. We could call our program "no pain, *all* gain."

Joan: All right. So let's introduce our program.

3

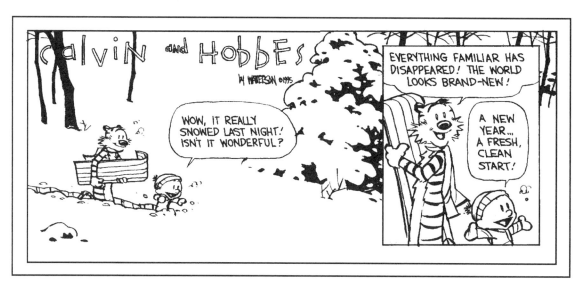

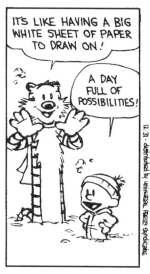

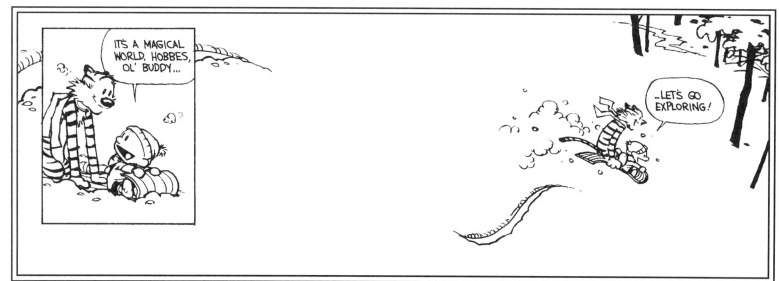

An Introduction to
Permanent Weight Loss

THE MISSING LINKS — **Nutrition**

The truth is, most weight-loss programs don't work. You know it, we know it. But now we know why they don't work. And one of the main reasons why they don't work is that they force us to deprive ourselves of something that is utterly natural to us—good-tasting food in adequate portions. Most of us have tried diet plans at one time or another. When we're on one of these plans, we usually manage to stick to it for a while . . . sometimes just a few days or a week . . . and sometimes for months. But during this time we know what we're missing: food that is really good, that has a satisfying texture and an attractive appearance.

We miss it. We crave it. Some of us even dream about it. If other family members are eating the foods we crave, we snitch pieces of it from their plates, or maybe from the leftovers when no one's looking. And sooner or later we return to the foods we want. If we've managed to lose any weight, we gain it right back—and then some. What happens to our self-esteem? We feel ourselves to be failures—we're not strong enough, not determined enough to lose weight.

In fact, depriving ourselves of tasty foods simply doesn't work.

Folks, we've been doing it all wrong. But now we know what does work.

For a start, the fat content of foods plays a leading role in making you fat or lean. One of the things we will show you in this book is how to track the amount of fat in various foods. Next, you'll learn about shopping smart; how to take the complexity out of the new food labeling, the kinds of foods to buy and the kinds to avoid. We'll follow that by describing how to eat smart—how to eat the kinds of foods that promote good health and keep our weight down while offering us delicious, satisfying meals.

One of the ways we'll do this is to show you how to substitute lower fat foods for higher fat foods, together with low fat cooking techniques that retain full flavor. With this knowledge, you'll be able to begin the process of *permanent* weight loss.

With the latest advances in research, we now know what is required for permanent weight loss; a whole series of links have to be in place before it works. These links aren't complicated or hard to do—you just have to learn what they are and how to do them. These are the links that have been missing from the dozens of diet plans you may have tried, and this is the reason these plans haven't worked.

Learning how to prepare and eat delicious, low fat meals, without depriving yourself, is one of the missing links of permanent weight loss.

Another missing link has to do with habits. Here we take a look at when and where we are tempted to overeat or eat the wrong things, including snack attacks. We show you how to eat smart at places where it's harder to maintain good eating habits, such as at the office, in restaurants, at parties, on trips, etc.

So get ready to discard many of your bad old eating habits and exchange them for new, healthier ones. *Good eating habits are another missing link of permanent weight loss.*

If you're a housekeeping mom, you know how much effort goes into caring for a family, and this includes meal preparation. After tending to blisters and bandages, tears and mends, homework, music lessons, laundry, etc., you dig deep into yourself for food creativity. When you plan family meals, you search for something your husband likes and that the kids will eat—something that can be prepared with ingredients you have on hand.

Guess who's last on the list? That's right, *you!* You're taking care of everyone's needs but your own. As you get left behind, so do your own food needs. And as long as you don't allow your own nutrition to be a high priority, you won't be eating smart. *So another of the missing links of permanent weight loss is learning how to take care of yourself.*

In this book you'll learn how to use daily reminders to keep your nutrition on the right track, you'll find wonderful recipes for pleasing your spouse and your kids, and they won't even know it's good for them (unless you tell them). You'll learn the smart way to use meat and you'll discover the truth behind the starch myth. You'll learn the secrets of "veggie power" and how to use fats selectively for flavor. *And you'll learn another missing link is that you can and should eat anytime you feel like it—but you'll learn to eat right.*

This is half of the story.

7

THE MISSING LINKS — **Fitness**

Let's say you're like most of us; as you get older, you tend to use your muscles less. And like most of us, you exercise when you can, but probably not often enough or regularly enough. Perhaps you've tried exercise programs in the past and found that the main result was aching muscles, or worse—boredom, boredom, boredom! And like the restrictive diet plans, after a while you stop exercising regularly or you quit completely.

So you're not getting enough exercise. What's the result of this? Over the long haul, it's a deterioration in your health. A short-term result is that you start to lose muscle mass; and as we'll explain later, the more muscle mass you lose from lack of exercise, the harder it will be for your body to eliminate excess fat. If you're not exercising regularly and you go on a restrictive diet, you will lose water and muscle, but only a little fat. Then when you go off the restrictive diet (as you eventually will), you'll most likely find that you're gaining weight even though you aren't eating any more than before the diet. In this book, we'll show you why that is and how to fix it.

One aspect of our program is that you won't pay much attention to your scale. This is because permanent weight loss is a result of achieving a higher level of fitness—not of counting pounds lost. In other words, as you become more fit, your body will lose excess fat until you are at the optimum weight for your size and build. You'll gauge your progress by your increasing fitness, and the fat loss will be automatic!

So here's another of the missing links: *you will lose weight permanently only as you become more fit.*

Great, you say, but what will help you stay on a fitness program when you know you should exercise more—and you don't?

We'll start by showing you, in this book, the effects of different kinds of exercises, and we'll describe how to achieve the right balance between them. Then we'll tell you about the common mistakes that many people make that cause exercise programs to be unpleasant or even unhealthy.

Exercising is a lot like eating. If food isn't satisfying, we don't eat it. And with exercise, if it's unpleasant or uncomfortable or inconvenient, we avoid it. *So another of the missing links to permanent weight loss is an ongoing fitness program that is enjoyable, convenient and effective.*

In this book, we'll show you how to create your own customized fitness program, and how to

- make it comfortable,
- make it convenient,
- make it fun.

But there are exercises and there are exercises. Not all have the same effect. So we'll give you the information that will

- make it work.

After we've shown you how to make exercise pleasant and effective, we'll describe another important point—how to develop a routine that is customized for you, a routine that you'll be able to continue indefinitely. Next we'll tell you how to

- make it last.

Getting Started

To help you get started on your own permanent weight loss, we've included a substantial number of outstanding low fat recipes that are easy to prepare and absolutely delicious—recipes that you will use over and over again. Once you become familiar with the low fat cooking techniques we describe, and the low fat substitutions we recommend, you'll be creating your own recipes. (Send them to us and we'll try to include them in our next edition!)

With the guides to fitness that we've provided, exercise drudgery is a thing of the past. You'll be able to create a fitness program that fits your schedule and your comfort level. And instead of guessing about the effects of exercise, now you'll know how to get the most out of it.

From all the advances in research over the past several years, we now have the knowledge of what is needed to achieve permanent weight loss and vital, exhilarating health. In this book you'll discover, in detail, the missing links that have made permanent weight loss so frustrating and elusive.

We now know that in order to achieve an optimum weight and maintain it, each link in the chain must be in place. In an easy, step-by-step process, we will show you each of these links so you can put them all together successfully.

The first section of our book covers the steps you will take to create your *food lifestyle*, and the second section shows you the steps needed to develop your *fitness lifestyle*. Combining all of these simple steps will help you achieve permanent weight loss!

9

Fat chance of that happening? More than a chance. This program works! You can say good-bye to restrictive diets that don't work and boring exercise programs.

You *can* achieve the permanent weight loss you've been wanting for so many years. We know. We've done it. What's more, you can do it in a way that adds zest and pleasure to your life.

Come on, join us. We invite you to get started—right now!

P.S. Before writing this book, we looked at many, many cooking, fitness and lifestyle books. Guess what? They're hard to read, the information is buried and scattered, and they don't explain what we really wanted to know. This book is different. Don't have time to read a chapter? Try one of our short, easy-to-read steps that take five minutes—they're simply packed with information that you have probably never seen before.

Skeptical? Okay, turn to Step 1 and read it. If you don't agree that this is the most enlightening thing you've ever read about weight loss, we'll . . . we'll . . . we're not sure what we'll do, but we'll do something!

Joan Cortopassi and Annette Cain

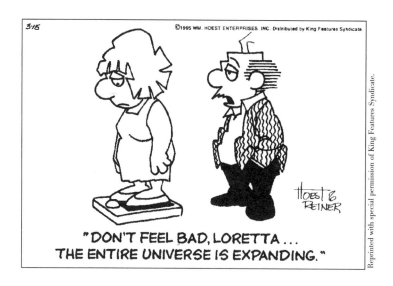

"DON'T FEEL BAD, LORETTA . . . THE ENTIRE UNIVERSE IS EXPANDING."

10

PART ONE

The Nature of Weight Loss

STEP 1 — A Revelation about Diets and Weight Loss

O kay, let's look at a typical situation. Clara B. is 5' 6" and weighs 156 pounds. Clara has a rather delicate frame, and for her size and body structure, she should weigh about 130. So she's some 26 pounds overweight.

Clara has tried eight—that's right, eight—different diet plans over the last several years. Some of them lasted for just a few weeks. One lasted for almost six months. None were much fun. Oh, the support from others in her dieting group was helpful, and it was nice to be able to talk about it with others in the same boat, but eventually, Clara's desire for tasty, satisfying food won out, just as it does with the rest of us. So she gave up on each of her diet plans and returned to her previous eating habits.

But wait! Something else happened. Each time she went off a diet plan and returned to her previous eating habits, she didn't just regain the few pounds she'd lost—she got even heavier. That is, after stopping a diet plan, Clara gained more weight and was heavier than before she'd started the plan.

Do you know anyone who's had this happen to them? Has it ever happened to you? What's going on here? Are imps playing tricks on us, or is it our karma causing us to become ever fatter?

Well, scientific research has solved the mystery, and in doing so, has given us valuable insight into how our bodies really work. So here's the answer to this puzzle.

If you read nothing else in this book— read this!

11

Calories are energy.

As you know, your body is a machine that takes in energy as food and expends energy as heat and movement and all the functions that keep you alive. And you know that if you eat more, the extra energy will either be worked off with more exercise or you'll get fatter. That's it—no way around it. So that's the energy balance of the body. Change either the amount of calories coming in or the amount of exercise, and you alter the balance—you get thinner or fatter.

Is that all there is to it? Let's look more closely and see.

Your body is composed mainly of muscle tissue, fat tissue, bone and water. While your bones are subject to change, they do so very slowly, so we'll skip them for the moment and look at muscle, fat and water.

Let's say you are living a rather sedentary life, without regular exercise, and your eating habits are fairly constant. You're consuming about the same number of calories month after month. Now, muscles need to be worked in order to maintain their size and vitality. Little or no exercise and they shrink. That's a very important point—so let's "note" it.

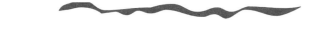

Okay, now remember the energy balance? If you continue to eat the same kinds of food you've been eating, and the small amount of exercise you're doing doesn't change, then your weight should stay the same. But if your muscles are slowly shrinking, how does your body compensate in order to stay at the same weight? Any guesses?

Muscles need to be worked to maintain their size and vitality.

You're right! It compensates by adding more body fat! Without adequate exercise, your body will compensate for its decreasing muscle mass by adding more body fat. So without an adequate exercise program, the proportion of fat to muscle

12

in your body will gradually increase. Now here's why this is so important. The only way your body can get rid of fat tissue is by chemically burning it off. Fat tissue can only be burned off by the working of muscles. Wow! That's also important enough to "note" by itself.

Fat tissue can only be burned off by the working of muscles.

So if you lose muscle mass because of lack of exercise, you lose the ability to burn off body fat. The more muscle you lose, the harder it will be for you to get rid of body fat.

Now let's say you go on a reduced-calorie diet, and you diet without a proper exercise program to go along with it. Now you've changed the energy balance—less energy coming in but everything else staying the same, so your body has to lose weight. But remember our dramatic statement in the box above; to paraphrase, the only way to get rid of body fat is by exercising. So if you're not exercising, your body has to lose weight somehow. Bones change very slowly, so that's out. What's left? Water and muscle. Your body needs some minimum amount of water to function, so after a few days of dieting, the water level in your body stabilizes. What's left for your body to reduce its weight? That's right—muscle.

So you continue on your diet for a while. Depending on the intensity of your diet, you lose a few pounds or many pounds of muscle. Then at some point you crave tasty food and you go back to your former eating habits. What happens next? Your body will quickly gain back the amount of weight that was lost, but it can't add muscle—remember, muscle can only be increased by exercise—so it can only do it by adding body fat. After you have quit your diet, you will not only be right back where you started, in terms of weight, but you'll have a higher proportion of body fat as well, and you'll have less muscle mass than before starting your diet.

Do you see what this means? You're off your diet and you're eating the same

13

> **"I'VE BEEN ON A DIET FOR TWO WEEKS AND ALL I'VE LOST IS TWO WEEKS."**
>
> —*Totie Fields*

as you did before you went on it—but now you have more body fat and less muscle mass. So even though you're eating the same as before, you will gradually put on *more* weight because there's less muscle to burn off your body fat.

That's why most of us keep gaining weight over the years even though we're not eating any more than we used to!

Now you see why exercise is so important to *permanent* weight loss. You can't lose weight permanently without adequate muscle mass to burn off body fat, and you won't have adequate muscle mass without exercising!

All right. Let's say you begin a good exercise program but your eating habits stay the same. Will this result in permanent weight loss? It depends on how much you're eating and how much you're exercising. For most of us, if we continue to eat a rich, high-calorie diet, a reasonable amount of exercise won't be enough to sustain permanent weight loss. And, as we'll see in the following sections of this book, most of our excess calories come from fat calories. But now let's say you combine a reasonable exercise program with a healthy, low fat, nutritional plan. Now you are attacking both ends of the energy balance: reducing caloric input and increasing your exercise output at the same time. The result is that your muscles increase and are able to burn off more fat tissue. From the combination of eating low fat foods and increasing muscle mass to burn off fat, excess fat is no longer created and stored in your body. The result? The proportion of fat in your body will be reduced to a level that promotes optimum health. We call this *fitness*.

14

Notice we haven't mentioned weight loss—yet. Now fitness is admirable for its own sake: when you're fit you feel better, have more energy, less illness, and you'll probably live longer. But here's another great benefit of fitness: when you reach a reasonable level of fitness, weight loss is an automatic side effect—a fantastic fringe benefit! So here's what we know.

1. **You will lose weight permanently only as you become more fit.**
2. **You will become more fit only by gaining more muscle, which burns more fat.**
3. **The only way to gain more muscle and burn more fat is through proper exercise, combined with healthy, low fat eating.**

15

So what do we know now? We know why most diets haven't worked, and why most of us have struggled to keep our weight down, without much success. But now we also understand what is happening. We know what to expect and we know how permanent weight loss can be achieved—only by the combination of smart exercise and smart eating.

So let's do it!

- **If your food energy intake is smaller than the total energy you use, you will have an energy deficit and weight loss.**

- **If your food energy intake is the same as the total energy you use, you will have an energy balance and maintain the same weight.**

- **If your food energy intake is larger than the total energy you use, you will have an energy surplus and weight gain.**

Everybody understands the above statements, but they're abstract. Let's place them in perspective. Eva weighs 140 pounds. She would like to lose about one pound of fat per week. What does she have to do in order to do that?

One pound of body fat has the energy value of 3500 calories. So in order to lose one pound per week, Eva has to burn up an extra 3500 calories each week. She can do that by eating less (especially eating less fat) and exercising more. How much does she have to reduce her fat intake and how much does she have to exercise? For the sake of simplicity, we'll assume that about half of her energy deficit will come from eating changes and half from exercise.

Let's further assume Eva is having a busy day and, for lunch, she has a fried chicken sandwich from a fast-food place. Her dinner includes an avocado salad. Later that night, she snacks on a large handful of peanuts (about ¼ cup). All of these are high fat, high calorie foods. The total fat content of these three food items provides about 250 calories of energy. To reduce her fat intake, let's say Eva substitutes a low fat sandwich for the fried chicken sandwich; she still has a tasty salad but without avocados; and she substitutes pretzels for the peanuts. By doing this she eliminates 250 fat calories from that day's calorie intake.

In committing to an exercise program, Eva feels that 30 minutes per day is too little but that she can't spare a whole hour, so she compromises on 45 minutes. She decides to begin her program by bicycling on a nearby bike

16

One pound of body fat has the energy value of 3500 calories.

path. Moderately paced cycling uses up about 335 calories per hour, so for her 45-minute effort, Eva uses up approximately 250 calories.

The 250-calorie food reduction plus burning 250 calories by exercise add up to a 500-calorie deficit per day. If Eva does this each day of the week, that's 500 calories x 7 days = a 3500-calorie deficit for the whole week.

> **You won't feel deprived by our program—you'll feel better, and you'll feel confident that, at last, a weight-loss program is really working for you.**

Now, back to where we began. One pound of fat has the energy value of 3500 calories. So by following this reduced fat/regular exercise program, she reduces her weekly caloric intake and increases her weekly caloric output to create a deficit of 3500 calories. Eva will lose the one pound per week that is her goal.

In later sections we'll show you the calorie and fat content of various foods. But for now, all we want to do is show you that an effective weight-loss program can be started without a lot of effort.

17

Eva didn't go on a boring, restrictive diet—what she did was a bit of smart nutrition planning and tasty substituting. True, it did take some changes in her scheduling to make time for her daily bicycling, but on the other hand, she did it with a friend and it was enjoyable and not overly taxing. Plus, she felt so energized by the exercise that she probably accomplished as much or more each day than she had before starting it.

And this is our whole point. You won't feel deprived by our program—you'll feel better, and you'll feel confident that, at last, a weight-loss program is really working for you.

Substituting tasty, lower fat foods for the avocado, the fatty chicken sandwich and the peanuts—hey, that's not too bad. Forty-five minutes of cycling on a pretty path with a friend? Why, that's downright pleasant. One pound of body fat gone each week? That's terrific!

STEP 3 — **Lowering Your Set Point**

Here's another helpful thing to know about achieving permanent weight loss—dealing with your body's set point.

You've probably noticed this at one time or another: you eat less for a time and maintain the same kinds of activities you have always done—but you don't lose weight. Why? What's happened is that your body doesn't like to change its weight, and it resists—by becoming more efficient. Scientists have shown that when we begin to lose weight, our body's metabolism actually slows down—we don't need as much food to sustain exactly the same activity as before. The effect is discouraging: we have reduced the amount of food we're eating and yet our weight remains the same.

> **One thing that changes your natural set point is lack of exercise.**

Actually, the same thing happens on the other end but it's usually not as noticeable because we don't pay attention to it. If we start eating more, our body compensates by raising its metabolic rate—that means it will burn up extra calories even though we aren't exercising more. So, for a while, we are able to eat more without gaining weight.

Each of our bodies has a tendency to remain at some constant weight—that weight is known as the body's *set point*. Why do some people have a naturally low set point and others a high one? No one knows. Perhaps your ancestors spent millennia trying to find enough food to survive, and your present-day,

18

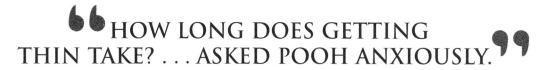

❝HOW LONG DOES GETTING THIN TAKE? . . . ASKED POOH ANXIOUSLY.❞

–*A. A. Milne*

inherited genes remember this and are insisting on a protective cushion—just in case. So your body responds by trying to stay at 150 pounds instead of the 125 pounds you would prefer.

High fat foods also tend to raise your set point.

Can your set point be changed? One thing that changes your natural set point is lack of exercise. As most of us age, our lifestyles change and we do less and less exercise over the years. This causes our set point to gradually drift upwards. And so we find ourselves stuck at ever-increasing weight levels, with our body resisting whenever we try to lose weight.

High fat foods also tend to raise your set point.

So if you combine healthy, low fat nutrition with regular exercise, can you lower your body's set point so that you are able to achieve permanent weight loss? The answer is yes. It's just that it takes a little longer for your body to adjust and adopt the new, lower set points as your weight begins to come down.

The purpose of bringing up the subject of set points is simply to alert you to the fact that, although you are doing everything right, it will take a while—perhaps months—before you actually begin to lose weight permanently.

But wait! Don't be discouraged. There is something you will start to lose more quickly. And it's in the next step.

19

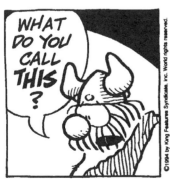
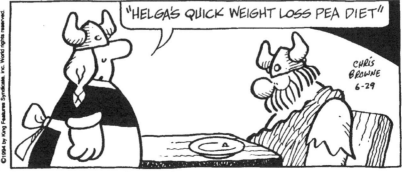

Reprinted with special permission of King Features Syndicate.

STEP 4 — Why You Should Throw Away Your Scale

(Or Hide It and Bring It Out Once Every Six Weeks)

Here's another mistake we've all been making in trying to lose weight—we've been weighing ourselves. Why is that wrong? Read on.

One difference between muscle and body fat is density. Muscle is three times as dense as body fat, and three times as heavy. Another way of looking at it is that muscle takes up only ⅓ the space of body fat. Got that? It's important enough to say it again.

Now let's look at why weighing ourselves will not tell us if we are progressing. From Step 1 we learned that a combined low

> **Muscle takes up only ⅓ the space of body fat.**

fat eating plan plus exercise program is necessary for permanent weight loss. And that the exercise builds muscle tissue, which burns more fat. So with this program, we're losing body fat and gaining muscle tissue.

Next, recall from Step 3 that our bodies have set points. That is, once you weigh a given amount for, say, several months or more, your body resists changing that weight.

Now let's set the scene and see what's happening. Marcus weighs 185 pounds. He looks overweight and feels heavy and sluggish. If we were to estimate, we would normally say he's about 25 pounds overweight. But instead, we're going to try a new approach. We're going to say he's several inches too thick—or that his waistline should be 32" rather than its present 38".

So Marcus has begun his C&T (Cook & Trainer) program. He is eating healthy, low fat meals and is exercising regularly. As a consequence, he is running a small energy deficit (fewer food calories ingested than are burned up), plus he is gaining muscle and losing body fat. But his body resists losing weight—it tries to stay at its set point of 185 pounds by becoming more efficient and needing fewer calories to

20

stay at the same weight. It can probably do this for anywhere from one to several months before losing weight.

But something else starts to happen more quickly. Marcus is staying at the same weight but is exchanging body fat weight for more muscle weight. Or you could say he's losing fat but gaining muscle.

Now remember, muscle takes up only ⅓ the space of body fat. Do you see what's happened? In exchanging body fat weight for more muscle weight, Marcus's body has gotten smaller—muscle takes up less space than body fat. So, in fact, Marcus's waistline will start to get smaller. He will look more trim and feel better, even though, for one or more months, he may not lose weight on the scale. Now bear with us while we repeat one more thing—from Step 1.

The proportion of fat in your body will be reduced to a level that promotes optimum health. We call this fitness. Notice we haven't mentioned weight loss—yet. Now fitness is admirable for its own sake: when you're fit you'll feel better, have more energy, less illness, and you'll probably live longer. But here's another great benefit of fitness: when you reach a reasonable level of fitness, weight loss is an automatic side effect.

21

When you start the C&T program, you will be paying attention to inches, not pounds. When we said "throw away your scale," we were just being dramatic. Actually, we recommend that you check your weight about once every six weeks. But stop the daily weighing—it will just frustrate you and sidetrack you from the more immediate benefits we will be monitoring. With our program, you will be losing inches where you want to lose them. So get ready to check out all those clothes that no longer fit.

Get ready to become more trim.

STEP 5 — **Fasting Isn't Lasting**

There are lots of theories about the virtues of fasting. Some claim fasting is good for eliminating toxins from the body, and some say it is a way of gaining spiritual insight; others state it's a good way to lose weight fast. But, from a permanent weight-loss standpoint, fasting is a no-no. Here's why:

When we drastically restrict the amount of food we eat, we are asking our bodies to run on empty. Being the wonderful machines they are, they are able to deal with this by switching into "red alert" or survival mode. This survival mode has some dire consequences.

1. When our bodies are not getting enough food energy (calories) they react by actually lowering the amount of energy they need.

2. The most efficient way to lower the amount of energy needed is to get rid of the tissue that requires the most energy to maintain.

3. Muscle tissue needs more energy to maintain than fat tissue. So our bodies go to work breaking down our muscles to lower the energy drain.

> **From a permanent weight-loss standpoint, fasting is a no-no.**

4. Fat tissue takes a tiny amount of energy to maintain so it is essentially left alone. Furthermore, since fat is easily stored, our bodies produce more fat-depositing enzymes which enable us to store as much fat as possible from what little food-fuel may be coming in.

Fasting can change your weight on the scale but, unfortunately, you lose the wrong kind of weight. Your body's survival mode has caused you to lose mostly muscle and water and very little fat.

Then comes a double whammy. You come off the fast and what happens next? You start putting the normal amount of fuel in your engine, but now your engine runs differently. Here's why. In Step 1 we said it is your muscles that burn fat. Now, when you were fasting, your body got into the survival mode and

22

tried to get rid of muscle because muscle needs more fuel to maintain. So what happened?

1. Now you have less muscle, which means less ability to burn fat.

2. And now you are putting the same amount of fuel into your body as before the fast.

3. But since you have less ability to burn fat, your body stores the extra energy as body fat.

4. Your body now has a huge work force of fat-depositing enzymes. In essence, you have become very efficient at storing fat, and it takes a long time to lay off all these workers.

So now, after your fast, you get back on the scale and notice that you've not only regained the weight you lost during the fast, you probably gained a few additional pounds as well. But the weight you regained is almost all fat! You now have more body fat than before you fasted and now you need fewer calories than before because you don't have as much muscle tissue.

The results of fasting are just the opposite of what you hoped for—after a fast, you're fatter than before and it is even harder than before to lose weight.

So from a permanent weight-loss standpoint, here's a word about fasting: *Don't!*

23

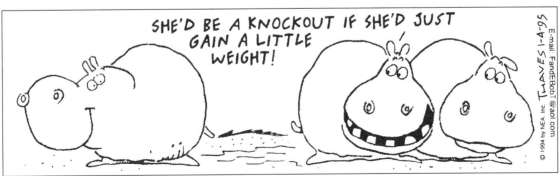

FRANK & ERNEST reprinted by permission of Newspaper Enterprise Association, Inc.

So far we've told you some things about the nature of weight loss . . . about how muscles burn body fat, about how the body's set point resists changes and why inches lost are initially more important than pounds lost, etc. Okay, fine. But how about actually doing it? What do you have to do to make it happen?

Three things. Track your fat intake, follow the Food Pyramid, and exercise regularly.

1. Fat Tracking

We'll tell you all about the fats in food. From this, you'll be able to determine how much fat you should be eating, how to track the fat in the things you do eat, and how to reduce your fat intake, without having to give up tasty, satisfying meals.

2. The Food Pyramid

Next we'll teach you all about the Food Pyramid, which is just a convenient symbol for showing you the kinds of foods you should eat, and in what proportions. You'll find that using the Pyramid makes planning meals for yourself and for your entire family easy and enjoyable.

3. Exercise

And lastly, we'll show you how to create an exercise program for yourself that is efficient, convenient, enjoyable, and that provides the fastest possible progress.

That's it! These *three* things will lead you to permanent weight loss, and they are all examined thoroughly in this book.

So get ready to learn everything you've ever wanted to know about losing weight and, more importantly, get ready to actually lose it and become healthier and more fit in the process!

24

PART TWO

Nutrition 101, Pass or Fail?

STEP 7 — **The Facts about Fats**

In this step we take a look at the different types of fats and the breakdown of unsaturated and saturated fats in various vegetable oils. We also look at where fat hangs out in all types of foods.

When we speak of fats in food, we are speaking of a type of fat called *triglycerides*. Almost all fats that we eat are triglycerides (95%); the other fats are phospholipids and sterols (5%). Triglycerides are the fats we are concerned with. They come in three forms, whose names are probably familiar to you:

Mono-unsaturated

Poly-unsaturated

Saturated

Mono-unsaturated fats are found in foods such as avocados, olives and olive oil, canola oil, almonds and ocean fish like salmon. With the exception of some fish, mono-unsaturated fats all come from plants. They are considered "good fats" because they reduce cholesterol levels in the blood. Poly-unsaturated fats are believed to be less beneficial but still pretty good. They are from safflower and sunflower oil, corn oil, walnuts and seeds. All poly-unsaturated fats come from plants. Saturated fats are the real culprits, for they have been shown to be related to a greater risk of heart disease and other problems of the cardiovascular system. The fat from animals is primarily saturated, as is fat from whole milk, butter, cheese and whole yogurt. In other words, all animal fat and all whole dairy fat is mostly saturated. In addition, a few plants yield saturated fat; the most common examples are coconut, palm and palm kernel oils.

Fat from animals is mostly saturated.

25

Food manufacturers also convert unsaturated fats to saturated fats by a chemical process. They do this in order to thicken or harden the vegetable oil within a food product, such as cookies or crackers. When fats of this kind are included in a product, they are called *hydrogenated*. Hydrogenated fats are artificially saturated fats, and they are as bad for you as naturally saturated fats.

The three kinds of triglycerides—mono-unsaturated, poly-unsaturated and saturated fat—all have the same amount of calories. So from a weight-loss standpoint, *ignoring other health concerns*, it doesn't make any difference what kind of fat you eat; what matters is *how much* fat you eat.

Some vegetable oils are more healthful than others and in the table below, the oils are listed from most healthful to least healthful. Notice, once again, that the highly mono-unsaturated oils are the most desirable and the highly saturated oils are the least desirable.

26

Types of Fat (in Grams) Per Tablespoon of Vegetable Oils

VEGETABLE OIL	MONO-UNSATURATED	POLY-UNSATURATED	SATURATED
OLIVE	12	1	2
CANOLA	10	4	1
PEANUT	8	5	2
SESAME	6	7	2
SOYBEAN	4	9	2
SUNFLOWER	3	11	1
CORN	3	10	2
WALNUT	2	9	4
COTTONSEED	2	9	4
PALM KERNEL	2	.5	12.5
COCONUT	1	.5	13.5

- **Mono-unsaturated fats are the most desirable type of food fats. Mono-unsaturated fats are always in a liquid state at room temperature.**

- **Poly-unsaturated fats are the next most desirable type of food fats. Poly-unsaturated fats are always in a liquid state at room temperature.**

- **Saturated fats, including hydrogenated fats, are the least desirable type of food fats. Saturated fats are usually thicker and are often solids at room temperature. Butter, margarine and lard are examples of saturated fats.**

How does the infamous *cholesterol* fit into this? Well, to begin, cholesterol isn't a fat; it's a kind of alcohol, a thick wax-like substance. Cholesterol has its good points. In fact, our bodies manufacture it to build cell membranes, nerve fibers and hormones. When we do eat foods that contain cholesterol, our body simply makes less of it. If we ingest too much cholesterol, it upsets the body's regulating mechanism and causes plaque to be deposited on the walls of blood vessels, leading to cardiovascular disease.

The same foods that contain a lot of saturated fat usually contain a lot of cholesterol. Examples are egg yolks, meats (especially organ meats) and whole dairy products; exceptions are coconut and palm oils. Only animal products contain cholesterol. So when we cut back on meats, eggs and whole dairy products, we automatically reduce our cholesterol intake.

Now back to the food fats—the triglycerides. Food fats are usually measured in two ways: calories and grams. You will be tracking the amount of fat you eat in terms of grams.

Only animal products contain cholesterol.

All three types of food fats—mono-unsaturated, poly-unsaturated and saturated— have the same number of fat grams and calories: about 5 grams of fat and 45 calories per teaspoon, and 15 grams of fat and 135 calories per tablespoon.

27

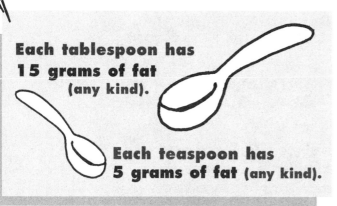

Each tablespoon has 15 grams of fat (any kind).

Each teaspoon has 5 grams of fat (any kind).

Daily Saturated Fat Intake

Remember, when we say that a type of fat is more or less good for you, we aren't talking about its calorie content, we're talking about your overall health. And in terms of health, we know saturated fats are the least beneficial. That's why we should try to keep saturated fats to a minimum. Since we recommend that 20% of your overall calories be from fat, 6.5% or less of your total fat should be saturated. Another way of saying this is that ⅓ or less of your total fat intake should be saturated fat. Example: your daily fat target is 33 grams. Your saturated fat target should be ⅓ of 33, or 11 grams of saturated fat per day maximum.

28

Daily Fat and Saturated Fat Targets

Your Daily Fat Target in Grams	Your Daily Saturated Fat Target in Grams
27	9
31	10
33	11
36	12
40	13
44	14
47	15
49	16
53	17
56	18
58	19
60	20
64	21
67	22
72	24
76	25

Besides the pure fat which we add to our food, fat occurs naturally in foods. How much fat is there in a cup of rice, a banana, a serving of Parmesan cheese, a serving of tofu? The following comparison tables will give you some idea of the fat content of a variety of foods.

Fat Content of Various Foods, by Food Group

BREADS/CEREALS/GRAINS STARCHY VEGETABLES & LEGUMES	PORTION	GRAMS OF FAT
Beans, cooked (all varieties)	½ cup	1
Bread	1 slice	1
Cereal	¾ cup	1
Rice, cooked	½ cup	1
Pasta, cooked	½ cup	1
Corn tortilla	1	1
Flour tortilla, whole	1	4 to 6
Flour tortilla, low fat	1	1
Barley/Oats/Rye, cooked	½ cup	1
Corn, cooked	⅓ cup	1
Potato, medium size	½	1
Bagel, plain	½	1
Graham cracker	2 lg. rectangles	1
Krusteaz pancakes	1 (4")	1
Gnocchi	2 ounces	1
Kavli	4 wafers	1
Smart Pop popped corn	3 cups	1
Pretzels, whole	1 ounce	1
Pretzels, nonfat	1 ounce	Trace
Tortilla chips	1 ounce	7
Low Fat tortilla chips	1 ounce	4
Low Fat potato chips	1 ounce	2 to 6
Rice cakes	2	1
Health Valley cookies	3 small	1
Soda crackers	4	1
Snackwell's crackers (wheat)	6	1

29

VEGETABLES	PORTION	GRAMS OF FAT
Most veggies	½ cup	Trace
Salad greens	1 cup	Trace
Tomato sauce	½ cup	Trace
Vegetable juice	½ cup	Trace
Salsa	½ cup	Trace

FRUITS	PORTION	GRAMS OF FAT
Banana	½	Trace
Grapefruit	½	Trace
Grapes	10	Trace
Fruit juice	½ cup	Trace
Melon	1 cup	Trace
Berries	1 cup	Trace

30

DAIRY PRODUCTS	PORTION	GRAMS OF FAT
Whole milk	1 cup	8
Low fat milk	1 cup	5
Light milk	1 cup	2.5
Nonfat milk	1 cup	Trace
Evaporated skim milk	1 cup	Trace
Buttermilk (low fat)	1 cup	2.2
Cream, heavy	½ cup	22
Whole ricotta cheese	1 cup	32
Nonfat ricotta cheese	1 cup	0
Whole cottage cheese	1 cup	10
Nonfat cottage cheese	1 cup	Trace
Whole sour cream	1 cup	40
Nonfat sour cream	1 cup	Trace
Ice cream, whole	½ cup	8 to 12
Ice milk	½ cup	3
Whole yogurt, plain	1 cup	16
Nonfat yogurt, plain	1 cup	Trace
Nonfat frozen yogurt	½ cup	Trace

Protein	Portion	Grams of Fat
Beans, cooked (all varieties)	½ cup	1
Eggs, whole	1	5 to 6
Egg whites	2	Trace
Egg substitute	¼ cup	Trace
Shrimp	1 ounce	Trace
Fish (firm, white meat)	1½ ounces	Trace
Salmon	1½ ounces	1 to 2
Chicken (breast meat), with skin	1¼ ounces	3 to 4
Chicken (breast meat), skinless	1¼ ounces	1 to 2
Tuna in oil	2 ounces	7 to 10
Tuna in water	2 ounces	1
Cheese, whole	1 ounce	8
Cheese, low fat	1 ounce	3
Cheese, Parmesan	2 tablespoons	3
Lean beef	1 ounce	3
Ground round	1 ounce	1 to 3
Lean pork (tenderloin)	¾ ounce	3
Tofu, raw, firm	¼ cup	5

Fats	Portion	Grams of Fat
Avocado	⅙	5
Butter/margarine	1 teaspoon	5
Vegetable oil, any	1 teaspoon	5
Mayonnaise, regular	1 teaspoon	5
Mayonnaise, low fat	1 teaspoon	1 to 2
Salad dressing, regular	1 tablespoon	5 to 10
Salad dressing, low fat	1 tablespoon	1 to 3
Olives, medium size	10	5
Peanuts, medium size	10 unshelled	5
Peanut butter	1 tablespoon	8
Tahini	1 tablespoon	8
Sunflower seeds, shelled	1 tablespoon	7
Bacon	2 pieces	6

31

The above comparisons are by food groups. Here's another way of looking at the fat content of foods—by grouping foods into low fat, medium fat and high fat foods.

Fat Content of Various Foods, by Grams of Fat per Average Serving*

FOODS WITH 0 TO 3 GRAMS OF FAT PER AVERAGE SERVING

All Fruit, except Avocado	Hard Candy	Jam and Jelly	Gumdrops
All Veggies	Most Breads	English Muffins	Jelly Beans
Bagels	Marshmallows	Most Cereals	Mustard
Potatoes	Catsup	Pretzels	Steak Sauce
Ryekrisp	Jell-O	Smart Pop Popped Corn	Sorbet
Pasta	Fruit Drinks	Rice	Egg Beaters
Beans	Egg Whites	Snackwell's Fat Free Cookies	Nonfat Dairy Products
Health Valley Cookies	Low Fat Tortillas	Nonfat Refried Beans	Fig Newtons
Bread Sticks	Fat-Free Salad Dressings	Graham Crackers	Saltines
Milk (1%)	Tuna (in Water)	Most Fish (Baked or Broiled)	

FOODS WITH 3 TO 5 GRAMS OF FAT PER AVERAGE SERVING

Low Fat Tortilla Chips	Chicken Breast (No Skin)	Low Fat Potato Chips	Turkey (White Meat)
Waffles/Pancakes (No Butter)	Clams	Sherbet	Low Fat Yogurt
Healthy Choice Frozen Dinners	Buttermilk	Low Fat Cottage Cheese	Low Fat Cheese
Avocado	Parmesan Cheese		

Average serving size is based on serving sizes used in the Food Pyramid and single serving sizes listed on food products.

32

FOODS WITH 5 TO 10 GRAMS OF FAT PER AVERAGE SERVING

All Beef	Breaded/Fried Fish	Lobster	Salmon
Chicken (w/Skin or Fried)	Cookies	All Pork	French Toast
All Lamb	Popcorn (Oil Popped)	Dark Turkey Meat	Puddings
Most Frozen Dinners	Milk Shakes	Low Fat Milk (2%)	Macaroni and Cheese
Tofu, Firm	Stuffing	Prepackaged Pasta Dinners	Granola
Feta Cheese	Regular Chips	Cream Cheese	Eggs
Regular Cheese	Sausage	Butter	Bacon
Margarine	Most Salad Dressings	Mayonnaise	Tahini
Miracle Whip	Crisco	Lard	All Oils (1 teaspoon)
Olives	Peanut Butter	Corn Nuts	

FOODS WITH MORE THAN 10 GRAMS OF FAT PER AVERAGE SERVING

All Nuts	Sunflower Seeds	Most Sauces	Trail Mixes
Ice Cream	Quiche	Pesto	Chocolate
Hot Dogs	Bologna (Including Turkey)	Shrimp Scampi	Most Fast Foods
Chili	Cakes	Candy Bars	Croissants
Doughnuts	Pizza	French Fries	Hash Browns

33

So now you have an idea of the fat content of various foods. Notice from the above tables that traditional American fare is loaded with fat. Every time you make your kids peanut butter sandwiches or use regular mayonnaise; every time you or your spouse douse your salad with regular salad dressing; every time you spread butter or regular cream cheese on your toast; every time you munch a hamburger or a piece of pizza; every time your favorite Mexican dish is topped with sour cream and guacamole—you are gulping huge doses of fat, much more fat than your body can possibly use.

Let's say that your daily fat target is 36 grams. A ham sandwich with mayonnaise, a handful of chips and a few fat-laden cookies—and that's your 36 grams of fat right there.

So what's left? Are all the good-tasting, yummy foods filled with fat? Is there no hope?

Don't despair. Remember what The Cook & The Trainer are all about—delicious, low fat food with no deprivation. In Parts 4 and 5 we will show you how to choose foods with a low fat content—and how to substitute tasty, lower fat foods for the high fat foods you may have been consuming.

Here are a few important points we'd like to remind you of about food fats:

34

- **Fats from plants are better for you than fats from animals and from whole dairy products.**

- **Hydrogenated fats are artificially saturated fats.**

- **All food fats have the same amount of calories.**

- **You're going to be tracking the amount of fat you eat in terms of grams.**

So there you have it—the facts about fats. In the next step we'll take a closer look at some fat fiction.

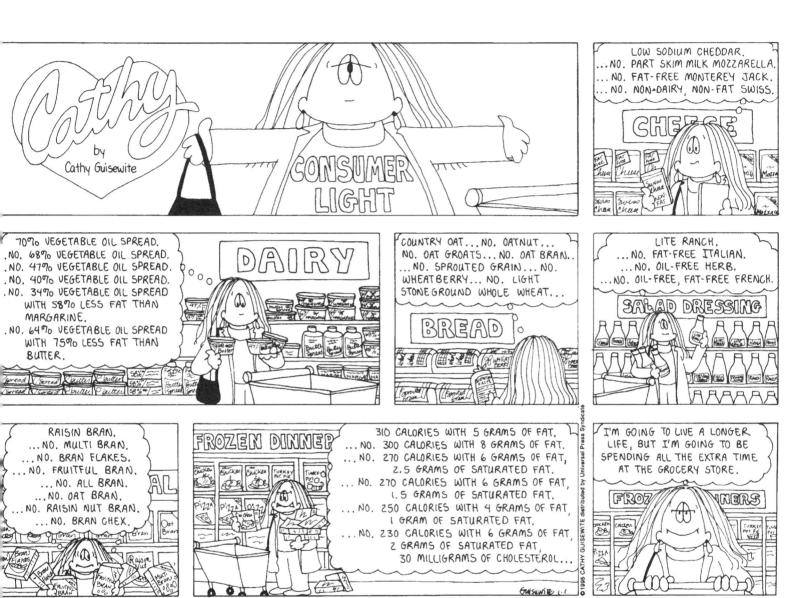

FAT CHANCE

STEP 8 — **97% Fat Free?**

You're in the grocery store and you see some hot dogs that claim they are 97% fat-free. You think to yourself, "Wow, this is too good to be true. A hot dog with only 3% fat in it!" So you toss them in your cart believing that they are 97% fat-free.

Well, unfortunately, this *is* too good to be true. There may be only 3% fat in the hot dog, but they mean 3% fat *by volume*, not by calories.

Here's another way of looking at it, using milk as an example.

Volume versus Calories

Type of Milk	"Fat Free" %	% Fat by Vol.	% Fat by Cal.	Fat Grams per Cup
Whole milk	97%	3%	37%	8
Low Fat milk	98%	2%	25%	5
Light milk	99%	1%	14%	2.5

So you can see that even though whole milk has only 3% fat by volume, in practical terms, a single cup of whole milk contains a large chunk of the total fat grams you should have each day.

The point we want to make in this step is simply this. There are two ways of measuring percentages of fat in foods: 1) by volume or weight, and 2) by calories. When you see a package of meat or dairy products that says something like "95% fat-free," they're measuring by volume to make you think there isn't much fat in it.

Now these claims of "92% fat-free" or "97% fat-free" written on a package don't come under the new labeling laws, so these labels can be misleading. But the new nutrition labels have to give you information in a more useable way.

And that's what the next step is all about—making sense of nutrition labels.

Food labeling was first introduced in the 1970s. It has come a long way since then, but even the new nutrition labels are overly complex and confusing. We'll take a look at a sample nutrition label and describe what it means, and then we'll show you which parts are most useful.

We have two explanations of nutrition labels: a very short one that is limited to the essential things you need to know for this permanent weight loss program, and a longer one, that explains everything on the labels. We'll give the short one first. You can read either one or both.

Nutrition Facts

1)	Serving Size: 2 cookies (24g)		
2)	Servings Per Container: 12		

		% Daily Value Calories
3)	**Calories:** 80	
4)	Calories From Fat: 52	

	Amount Per Serving	% Daily Value Calories
5)	**Total Fat** 6g	**9%**
6)	Saturated Fat 4g	6%
7)	**Cholesterol** 0 mg	**0%**
8)	**Sodium** 90 mg	**4%**
9)	**Total Carbohydrate** 20g	**7%**
10)	Dietary Fiber 1g	4%
11)	Sugars 12g	—
12)	**Protein** 1g	—

Very Short Explanation of Nutrition Labels

Here's an example of a typical label for a box of cookies. For tracking your daily calories, you need to look at lines 1 and 3; for tracking your daily fat intake, you need to look at lines 1, 5 and 6.

Line 1: Serving size. Is 2 small cookies a reasonable serving size? Not for most of us. So how many cookies are you going to eat? Four? Six? Twelve? Let's say you're not going to OD and you'll limit yourself to 6. That's three times as many as the manufacturer's serving size. So you'll need to multiply all their figures by 3.

Line 3: In our program the emphasis is on counting daily fat intake. Nevertheless, calories certainly do exist, and if you ingest a humongous amount of them, you'll gain weight no matter how little fat you eat. A good rule of thumb is to limit the calories in any serving of a dish

37

to 100 or less—that way your total calorie intake won't get out of hand. Note that these particular cookies are highly caloric; six cookies equal 240 calories!

Line 5: Their total fat of 6 grams, multiplied by 3, equals 18 grams of fat. If you eat those six cookies, you're going to gobble 18 grams of fat (which is a big chunk of your daily allotment).

Line 6: Most of the fat in these cookies is saturated fat. If you eat six cookies, multiply their figure of 4 grams of saturated fat by 3 which equals 12 grams of saturated fat. Remember that we (and most health authorities) recommend that ⅓ or less of your total fat intake should be saturated. These cookies definitely don't offer that; six cookies have 12 grams of saturated fat out of a total of 18 grams of fat which is about ⅔, or 67% saturated fat.

So you have to make a decision. Find some tasty nonfat cookies to replace them, or go ahead and eat them, but make sure that the rest of the fat you eat on this particular day is unsaturated.

Anyway, that's all you need to know about the nutrition labels to track your daily calories and fat: the size of the serving you intend to eat, and the total number of calories, fat grams and saturated fat in your serving.

Complete Explanation of Nutrition Labels

First of all, you may notice that some of the items on nutrition labels are printed in bold type and some are not. The bold type items are mandatory; food manufacturers must list them. Other listings are optional.

Line 1: Most of the figures on nutrition labels are based on the serving size, and the manufacturer gets to say what a serving is. Some manufacturers give a realistic serving size, but many don't. In the case of the label example on the following page, the only one who will eat a mere 2 small cookies is your pet hamster. So first of all, look at the serving size on a label and determine if it's a reasonable amount for you. If not, you'll have to multiply all the figures on the label by how

38

Nutrition Facts

		Amount Per Serving	% Daily Value Calories
1)	Serving Size: 2 cookies (24g)		
2)	Servings Per Container: 12		
3)	**Calories:** 80		
4)	Calories From Fat: 52		
5)	**Total Fat** 6g		**9%**
6)	Saturated Fat 4g		6%
7)	**Cholesterol** 0 mg		**0%**
8)	**Sodium** 90 mg		**4%**
9)	**Total Carbohydrate** 20g		**7%**
10)	Dietary Fiber 1g		4%
11)	Sugars 12g		—
12)	**Protein** 1g		—

much you increase the serving size. Example: you decide that 6 cookies, rather than two, is a reasonable amount. Then Line 5, total fat per serving, becomes 6 grams of fat multiplied by 3, which means that you're eating 18 grams of fat with your 6 cookies.

For the remainder of the figures in this label example, we'll assume that the serving size is six cookies.

Line 2: Number of servings per container. The label says 12 servings at 2 cookies per serving, which means there are 24 cookies in the package. At 6 cookies a whack, that's only 4 servings.

Line 3: Calories really means calories per serving. If you're tracking your daily calorie intake, multiply their 80 calories per serving by 3, which means 240 calories per serving of 6 cookies.

Line 4: If you're tracking calories, 52 calories of fat per serving out of a total of 80 calories per serving is a lot of fat. Multiply the 52 fat calories by 3 and you have 156 calories of fat for 6 cookies.

Line 5: There are two items on this line: in this example, there are 6 grams of fat per serving and they contribute 9% to your total calorie intake. The grams-of-fat figure is useful, but the percentage figure is based on a total daily intake of 2000 calories with 30% of total calories from fat. Since not everyone is eating 2000 calories, and since we (and most health authorities) recommend a lower percentage of fat than 30%, the percentage figures on labels are not very useful.

For our example, remember to multiply the 6 grams of fat by 3 to give 18

39

grams of fat for the six cookies you're eating. If your total daily allotment of grams of fat is, say, 38, then 18 grams of fat for these little cookies is a lot.

Line 6: The example above shows 4 grams of saturated fat that contribute 6% to your total calorie intake. The first figure is useful. Remember that it's for two cookies only. If you're having six cookies, multiply the 4 grams by 3, which equals 12 grams of saturated fat. Compare this 12 grams of saturated fat to the 18 grams of total fat from Line 5; 12 over 18 is ⅔, or 67% of the fat in these cookies is saturated. Remember, ⅓ of your total fat intake or less should be saturated. So you have to decide whether to substitute some tasty nonfat cookies for these or, if you still want them, make sure that the rest of your fat on this particular day is unsaturated.

As with the percentage figures on the other lines, the percentage figure on this line is only for a 2000-calorie, 30% fat diet.

Line 7: If you're tracking your daily cholesterol intake, the first figure—milligrams of cholesterol per serving—can be useful, but once again, the percentage figure is based on 2000 calories, 30% of them from fat, which is not what we'll be doing.

Line 8: If you're on a limited-salt diet, this first figure, in milligrams (1/1000 of a gram), is useful. It's based on a total daily salt intake of 2250 milligrams. So if you're tracking salt intake, you'll have to adjust the percentage figure to fit whatever your personal daily salt intake is.

Line 9: The total carbohydrate amount isn't very useful because it doesn't distinguish between complex carbohydrates (the healthy ones) and simple carbohydrates (refined starches and sugars). The percentage figure is based on a total daily carbohydrate intake of 286 grams.

Line 10: Dietary fiber in grams can be useful if you're tracking your total daily fiber intake. The percentage figure on this line is based on a total daily fiber intake of 25 grams.

Line 11: If you're tracking or trying to limit sugar, this figure can be helpful.

A teaspoon of sugar equals 5 grams of carbohydrate. Divide the total grams of sugar by 5 to give you the number of teaspoons per serving. Remember to multiply it by 3 for a serving of 6 cookies. No percentage of total diet is given for sugar because no standards for total sugar intake have been set.

Line 12: As adults, we don't need much protein to be healthy. In fact, most of us eat too much protein. So this figure can be useful to limit your total daily protein intake.

Ingredients

Ingredients on food labels are always listed by weight, starting with most and ending with least. If a food lists a fat as one of its first ingredients or if it lists several high fat ingredients (butter, cheese, cream, etc.), then it is most likely a high fat food. The same goes for sugar. This additive is abundant in most processed foods and is often hidden behind words like corn syrup, barley malt, fructose or cane juice. It is important to look at the ingredients to see how wholesome the food is. Try to avoid products with a lot of additives and preservatives. A good rule of thumb is: the more unpronounceable ingredients there are, the less wholesome the food is.

> **A good rule of thumb is: the more unpronounceable ingredients there are, the less wholesome the food is.**

41

Interpreting the Terms and Claims on Food Labels

In general, the formal nutrition labels that we described above are the most accurate indicator of what's in a product. However, the food industry employs a number of additional terms which only create consumer confusion. But if you know what they mean, they can help you figure out the product's real contents. The following are the terms commonly used.

LABEL CLAIM	DEFINITION
Calorie Free	Less than 5 calories per serving
Low Calorie	40 calories or less per serving
Reduced Calorie	At least 25% fewer calories than normal
Light or Lite	Product has at least 1/3 fewer calories or 50% less fat; if more than half the calories are from fat, fat content must be reduced by 50% or more
Fat Free	Less than 0.5 gram of fat per serving
Low Fat	3 grams of fat or less per serving
Reduced Fat	At least 25% less fat than normal
Less Fat	Example: "Reduced fat brownies - 25% less fat than our regular brownies." Meaning: fat content has been reduced from 8 to 6 grams per serving.
Lean	Meat, poultry, seafood and game meat with less than 10 grams of total fat, less than 4 grams of saturated fat, and less than 95mg of cholesterol per reference amount.
Extra Lean	Meat, poultry, seafood and game meat with less than 5 grams of total fat, less than 2 grams of saturated fat, and less than 95 mg of cholesterol per reference amount.

42

Reminder

Remember, the quick way to track fat from nutrition labels is to:

• Look at the serving size on the label and decide what is a reasonable serving size for you. Is it the same as theirs, is it two times as large or three times as large?

• Multiply the grams of fat per serving on the label by how much larger your serving size is. That's the grams of fat you'll be consuming. Compare this to your daily fat target in grams.

• Multiply the grams of saturated fat per serving on the label by how much larger your serving size is. That's the grams of saturated fat you'll be consuming. Total daily saturated fat should be ⅓ of your total daily fat intake (of all kinds) or less.

• If you are tracking your total calories, multiply the number of calories per serving by how much larger your serving is. That's the number of calories you'll be consuming.

(The definitions of label terms and claims are from Label Facts for Healthful Eating, *published by the National Food Processors Association.)*

Whaт are starches? The whitish, sticky stuff in foods that is satisfying to eat and which makes you fat? Well, yes and no. To understand what starches are, you have to know starch is a carbohydrate and then remember there are two types of carbohydrates: complex and simple. Complex carbohydrates are found in grains, seeds, beans, fruits and veggies. Simple carbohydrates are *all* sugars.

Starch is a complex carbohydrate; it is the main form of carbohydrate in almost all plants. Most of the starch in our diet comes from bread, pasta, rice, corn and potatoes. In contrast, celery, lettuce, broccoli and tomatoes contain essentially no starch. Among fruits, bananas are high in starch, while grapes, melons and peaches are starch-free.

Starch, *in its natural form as a complex carbohydrate*, is good for you because it combines fuel for your body with health-promoting vitamins, minerals and fiber. Complex carbohydrates keep your blood sugar stable because, unlike simple sugars, they are absorbed into the bloodstream *slowly*. This helps your body to stay in chemical balance. They also signal your brain that you have had enough to eat. This, together with the slow absorption, gives you a longer period of feeling full and a sense of well-being.

The more that natural starch is processed, the less nutritious it becomes. For example, white bread has been processed to the point where most of the vitamins, minerals and fiber have been eliminated—what is left is almost pure, refined starch. Also, in many plants, vitamins and minerals are concentrated in the skins and husks, so that when these are removed, as with potatoes and rice, much of

43

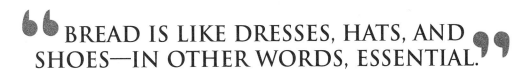

❝BREAD IS LIKE DRESSES, HATS, AND ❞ SHOES—IN OTHER WORDS, ESSENTIAL.
–Emily Post

the nutritional value is lost. Processed carbohydrates are a double whammy—not only are nutrients lost, but fats, artificial stabilizers, sugar and salt are usually added as part of the processing.

> **Complex carbohydrates give you a longer period of feeling full and a sense of well-being.**

There is a big difference between processing and cooking. Processing strips away nutrients and adds undesirable substances to the food. Cooking complex carbohydrates, in contrast, is often beneficial. Not only do they taste better after being cooked properly, they are also easier to digest. For example, if you eat rice or pasta raw, most of the nutrients will pass through your body undigested.

There is also a big difference between simple and complex carbohydrates. Simple carbohydrates are naturally and chemically refined sugars, such as honey, molasses, corn syrup, maple syrup and white and brown sugar. Sugars don't signal the brain that we are full—that's one reason why many of us are tempted to overeat sweets. Sweet foods don't contain as many calories as fatty foods, but for many health reasons, they should be eaten in moderation.

Refined sugar, found in our modern confections, doesn't occur in nature, and our bodies are not built to handle it very well. Refined sugars are digested swiftly

44

> **"PRAY FOR PEACE AND GRACE AND SPIRITUAL FOOD, FOR WISDOM AND GUIDANCE, FOR ALL THESE ARE GOOD, BUT DON'T FORGET THE POTATOES."**
> —*John Tyler Pettee*

after being eaten and they raise our blood sugar to abnormal levels, upsetting the body's chemical balance. If you eat a large portion of candy, cookies, ice cream, etc., your body reacts by releasing insulin, which tries to return your blood sugar to a normal level. To do this, insulin will convert any *excess* sugar to *fat!*

Processed starches like white bread, white rice and packaged pastas are digested in much the same way as refined sugars because they no longer have the nutrients (vitamins, minerals, fiber) to be absorbed more slowly by the body. Eating *large amounts* of processed starches will increase the amount of sugar that gets converted to fat. So when you eat lots of sugar and processed starches, not only are you ingesting calories quickly, you are also putting a lot of strain on your body to stay balanced.

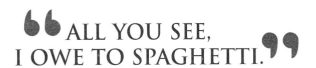

ALL YOU SEE, I OWE TO SPAGHETTI.

–*Sophia Loren*

45

Nutritional science has come a long way in recent years. Twenty years ago we were supposed to limit our starches because we were told they would make us fat. Well, of course, if you regularly eat three times the normal portion of a starch—especially processed starch—the huge amount of calories *will* increase your weight. But, by and large, the old myth isn't true. It's not starches that make us fat—it's the fat things we put on top of them or mix with them that make us fat. As examples, notice the following comparisons:

LOW FAT		HIGH FAT
Spaghetti w/marinara	vs.	Fettuccine Alfredo
Brown rice	vs.	Risotto with cream and cheese
French bread	vs.	Garlic bread w/butter or oil
Whole wheat bagel w/nonfat yogurt	vs.	Bagel w/regular cream cheese

How you prepare complex carbohydrates also determines their fat content. In the steps on low fat cooking techniques, we'll show you how to prepare complex carbohydrates so you get lots of flavor with a minimum of fat.

A Brief Review

Since the majority of your food-fuel will come from complex carbohydrates, it's important to know the differences between simple and complex carbohydrates.

Simple carbohydrates are refined sugars—eat them in moderation. In large amounts, they cause chemical imbalances in the body and provide little or no overall nutritional benefit.

Complex carbohydrates consist of all unprocessed grains, vegetables and fruits. Processing robs these foods of much of their nutritional value.

Starches are the main component of complex carbohydrates. In their unprocessed form, starches are combined with fiber, vitamins and minerals and are very beneficial to good health.

Starches, by themselves, don't make you fat *when eaten in moderate amounts*—it's the fats that you cook them in or serve with them that make them fattening. So watch out for the company they keep!

46

STEP 11 — **How about Supplements?**

Supplements have probably been controversial since the first vitamins were able to be isolated and manufactured separately from food. The basic scientific question has been: are vitamins, minerals and other supplements beneficial to us if we are eating a normal, balanced diet? After many years of research and testing, there is still no absolutely clear answer that applies to everyone.

It's beyond the scope of this book to take sides on this general argument, but there are a few well-established facts about food supplements. We present them here.

We know our bodies need certain vitamins and minerals in order for us to avoid illness. And after many years of testing, our public health agencies know the minimum amounts of each of these vitamins and minerals that are necessary to avoid certain ill-

> ❝ VITAMIN ADS ARE SO ATTRACTIVE, THEY MAKE A MAN WHO HAS HEALTH FEEL LIKE HE'S MISSING SOMETHING. ❞
>
> *–Evan Esar*

nesses. In theory, all of these necessary vitamins and minerals are present in the foods we eat, if we have a nutritious, well-balanced diet. If, for some reason, the essential vitamins and minerals are lacking in the food we eat, it is necessary to supplement our diet with additional vitamins and minerals to avoid vitamin-deficiency illnesses.

This is accepted—no controversy about it. Yet, there is a great deal of controversy (and hype) about some other aspects of vitamin and mineral supplements. We will try to address these issues here:

Q: **Should I take vitamin and/or mineral supplements?**

A: While there is evidence to show that vitamin and mineral supplements do benefit some people, it's impossible to say for sure which individuals will benefit.

47

In general, most health authorities regard modest doses of vitamin and mineral supplements as added insurance for good health, as long as they are not used as a substitute for a nutritious, well-balanced diet.

Q: Is it harmful to take more than the minimum recommended doses of vitamins and minerals?

A: Some vitamins and minerals are toxic in large dosages. The maximum doses for these have been set by government health agencies. Commercially available supplements limit the amounts of all potentially toxic vitamins and minerals to these maximum amounts.

48

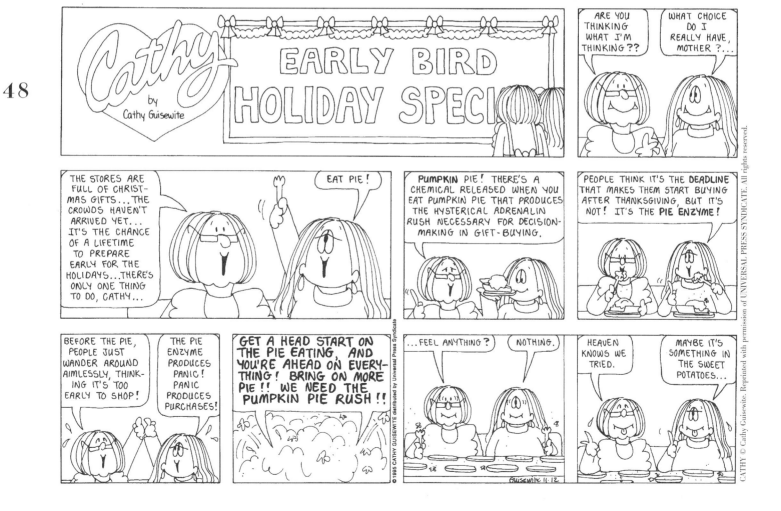

Q: With the exception of the potentially toxic vitamins and minerals, is it beneficial to take more than the minimum recommended doses?

A: Nobody knows for sure. The minimum recommended doses have been established on the basis of avoiding certain diseases in the average person. What is controversial is whether or not higher-than-minimum levels of vitamins and minerals can improve our health beyond the mere avoidance of certain diseases.

Q: Is it true that vitamin and mineral supplements help to prevent some diseases, including cancer and heart disease?

A: There is increasing evidence to show that this is true for a population group as a whole. For example, if you divide 10,000 people in half and give supplements to one of the groups, but not to the other, the group receiving the supplements might have 100 fewer cases of some diseases and that group, overall, might live longer. Would *you* be one of those 100 persons saved from illness or given greater longevity if you took supplements all your life? No one knows.

Q: Is it true that following the guidelines of the nutritional pyramid, and eating a range of fresh, healthy foods can keep you healthier and make you live longer?

A: A few people can thrive on poor diets, and there have been centenarians (those who have lived 100+ years) who claim to have smoked a cigar and drunk a bottle of whiskey every day of their adult lives. But for most of us, the evidence is clear that a proper diet does keep us healthier longer.

Q: Why can't vitamin and mineral supplements make up for a poor diet?

A: There are trace amounts of chemical compounds (e.g. phytochemicals and antioxidants) in natural foods that have not even been isolated yet. In other words, no manmade supplement, so far, contains all the trace elements that occur naturally in foods. In addition, vitamins and minerals cannot supply the

49

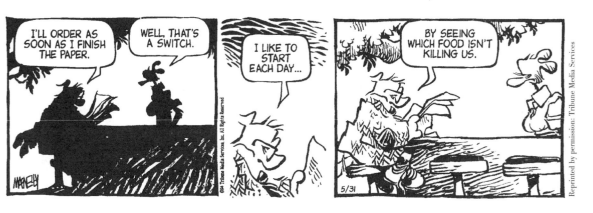

fiber, balanced protein and other essential factors that are present in natural foods.

Q: Aren't there special circumstances where supplements are needed?

A: There are circumstances where individuals *may be more likely* to need nutritional supplements. These include vegans (those on a vegetarian diet with no dairy products), pregnant women, athletes in training, dieters eating less than 1500 calories per day, and individuals with food allergies, such as lactose intolerance. Also, vitamin and mineral requirements may increase for elderly people.

Q: There has been a lot of publicity over the years about megadoses (very large amounts) of vitamin supplements. Are these beneficial, or can they be harmful?

A: There is increasing statistical evidence to show that megadoses of some vitamins, such as Vitamin C, Vitamin E and Beta Carotene are beneficial. Extensive research is needed for more concrete evidence of the effects of vitamin megadoses.

Q: Isn't it true that vitamins and minerals must be taken in balanced amounts—that is, a certain amount of one vitamin with a certain amount of another?

A: It's true. When certain vitamins are taken in combination with other vitamins and minerals, they help each other get absorbed better. Fortunately, essentially all commercially available *combination* vitamin/mineral supplements are correctly balanced.

Q: What about weight loss pills, appetite suppressants, etc.?

50

A: The answer to this reflects our personal bias. We recommend you avoid them. It is our belief that the farther away you get from a natural diet, the more health problems you are courting. We do think it's ironic that all diet pill and weight loss schemes recommend you eat low fat foods and exercise regularly as part of their regimen.

Q: What about sugar and fat substitutes?

A: Again, the answer to this reflects our personal bias. We believe the most nutritious and healthy foods are ones that are all-natural and wholesome. Remember, for the most part, fat and sugar are items we add to our foods and we should eat them sparingly. If you are using moderation, you don't have to worry about the calories and fat, so use the real thing. Eating fake fats will only increase your chances for health problems. Although studies have shown that sugar substitutes and natural gums are safe when used in moderation, why not have the real thing—sugar and fat—in moderation?

Q: So what should I do?

A: Eat a proper diet that includes a wide variety of fresh, unprocessed foods. If you are in special circumstances where you are more likely to need a supplement, or if you want additional protection, choose a *combination* vitamin/mineral supplement (as opposed to a high dose of one particular vitamin, protein powders or other artificial nutrients). Try to use good-quality supplements (i.e., all natural; without artificial fillers, colors, binding agents, etc.).

We ourselves take a good-quality vitamin and mineral supplement once every few days.

51

CAUTION

This step is provided as general information. It is not intended to replace sound medical advice and it may not be beneficial for your particular condition and circumstances.

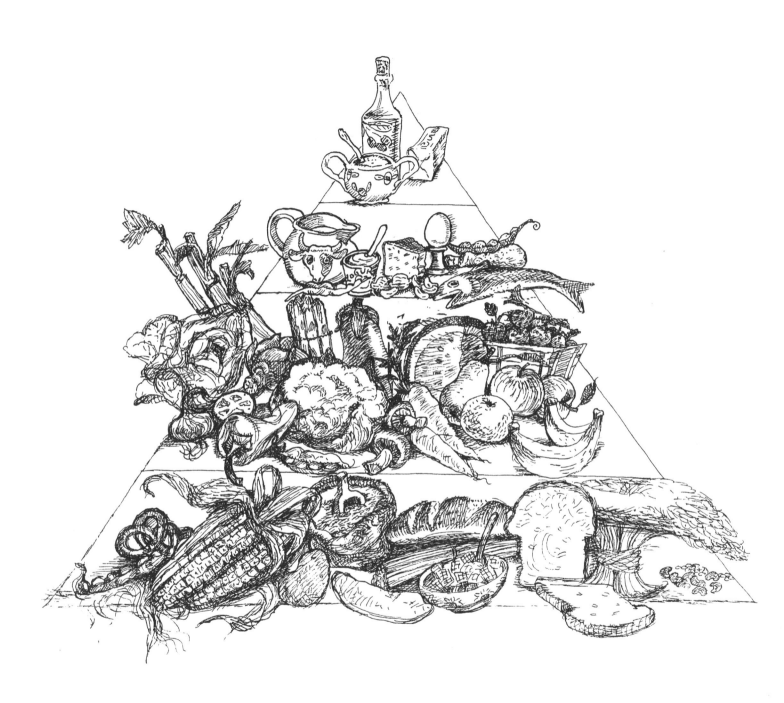

PART THREE

Pyramid Power

STEP 12 — **The Building Blocks**

The Six Types of Essential Nutrients

1. **Carbohydrates**
2. **Fat**
3. **Protein**
4. **Vitamins**
5. **Minerals**
6. **Water**

Many of us have heard the saying, "You are what you eat." It's true—our diet does affect our health. We need to fill up with high-quality fuel to get the best performance from our bodies. If you are dieting or are following a nutritional plan, you need to make sure you are getting the right kinds of nutrients in adequate amounts. This step briefly reviews some nutrition basics.

To plan and cook healthy, well-balanced meals it is important to know what kind of fuel your body needs and which kinds of foods that fuel comes from. Food is a fuel composed of six types of nutrients which are essential for maintaining optimal health and fitness. These nutrients are described below.

Carbohydrates

There are two types of carbohydrates: complex and simple. Complex carbohydrates are found in whole grains (brown rice, multigrain breads and cereals), beans, fruits and veggies. Simple carbohydrates are from sugars and refined starches (like white bread).

53

Complex carbohydrates are the best choice for fueling your body.

Complex carbohydrates are the best choice for fueling your body. This is so because they contain large amounts of vitamins, minerals and fiber and are absorbed slowly into your body. This slow absorption is very important; it enables your body to stay in nutritional balance. Simple carbohydrates, in contrast, contain essentially no vitamins, minerals or fiber—they are empty calories. And because they are absorbed very quickly by your body, they cause drastic changes in blood sugar levels which, in turn, upset your body's delicate chemical balance. *One gram of carbohydrate has 4 calories.*

Fat

Fat is a very concentrated source of food energy. In other words, fat has lots of calories. *One gram of fat has 9 calories.* We all need a small amount of fat in our diet in order to absorb fat-soluble vitamins (A, D, E and K). Fat also plays an important role in hormone and cell functioning and provides a physical cushion for internal organs. Fat comes from animal sources (butter, lard, meat, fish) and vegetable sources (nuts and plant oils, such as peanut, corn, olive oil, etc.).

Protein

Protein is the only nutrient which builds and repairs muscle, red blood cells, hair and other tissues. Because protein's main job is to build and repair tissue, it is not a primary source of food energy for the body. However, the body will use it for fuel if not enough calories are available (starvation diet or exhausting exercise). Many protein-rich foods are also rich in fat, so you must choose protein wisely. Low fat protein sources include egg whites, fish, lean poultry, beans, low fat cheese and nonfat dairy products. *One gram of protein has 4 calories.*

Vitamins and Minerals

Vitamins and minerals are not sources of food energy (calories). They are nutrients that are necessary in small quantities to enable the body to perform its complex functions. Some of the commonly known vitamins are A, B complex, C, D and E.

54

While our bodies can manufacture some vitamins, most of them must be obtained from a well-balanced diet. Some of the minerals essential to good health are calcium, magnesium, phosphorous, potassium, sodium and zinc. Minerals are obtained exclusively from the foods we eat. Most vitamins are either diminished or destroyed by overcooking. Minerals are heartier and do not deteriorate during cooking.

Water

Water does not provide food energy, but it is an essential nutrient that makes up more than half our body weight. Water provides the medium in which nearly all of the body's

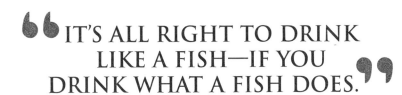

IT'S ALL RIGHT TO DRINK LIKE A FISH—IF YOU DRINK WHAT A FISH DOES.

—Mary Petitbone Poole

55

activities are conducted. Some of its primary functions include stabilizing body temperature, transporting nutrients to cells and waste away from cells, and helping with metabolism. Depending on your body weight, you should drink eight to ten 8-ounce glasses of water or liquid each day—more if you are exercising a lot or if you are in a hot environment. Does it have to be plain water? Not necessarily, but you need to be aware of a few things: caffeinated coffee, tea and soda have a dehydrating effect on the body, so you are defeating the purpose of drinking water if your total liquid intake consists of coffee, tea and/or soda. Also, you need to be aware of the extra calories you are taking in with other drinks, especially sodas sweetened with sugar, and sweetened fruit juices and fruit drinks. So for optimum health and to keep your caloric intake down, choose water as often as possible.

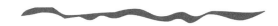

In the next step, you'll learn how these essential nutrients—the building blocks—are translated into the Food Pyramid.

56

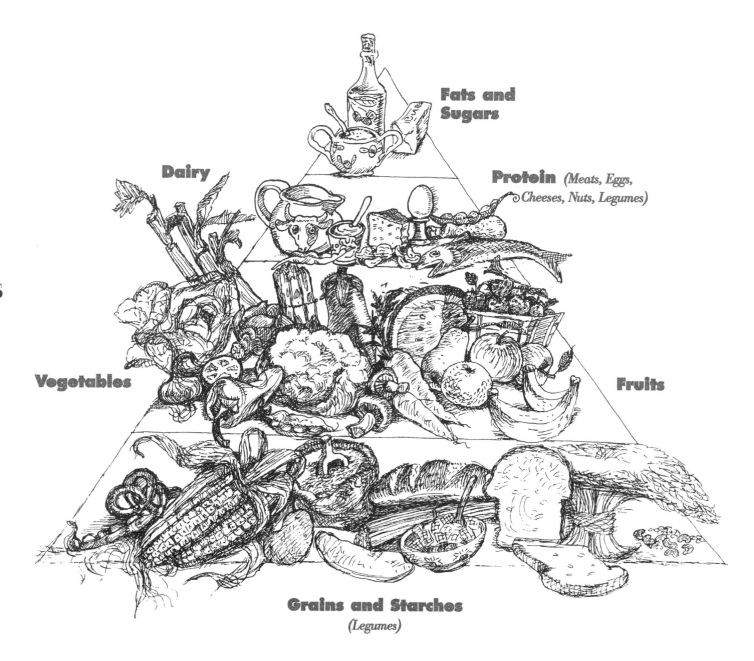

Fats and Sugars

Dairy

Protein (*Meats, Eggs, Cheeses, Nuts, Legumes*)

Vegetables

Fruits

Grains and Starches

(*Legumes*)

The Pyramid is a model of what to eat each day. It's not a right prescription, but a general guide that lets you choose a healthful diet. It separates all kinds of foods into food groups and tells you which food groups you should eat more of and which you should eat less of. By following this general guide, you will be eating a well-balanced, healthy diet that helps you lose weight and keep it off.

There are six sections and four levels within the Pyramid. The choice of a pyramid shape is deliberate. Notice the lower levels are considerably larger than the upper levels. This is to indicate that, for good health, you need to eat larger amounts of the foods from the lower levels and smaller amounts of food from the higher levels. The Pyramid's six sections represent the six major food groups:

- **Fats and Sugars**
- **Dairy Products**
- **Proteins (Meats, Eggs, Cheeses, Nuts and Legumes)**
- **Vegetables**
- **Fruits**
- **Grains and Starches (Legumes)**

The Pyramid emphasizes foods from the three lower levels. Each of these food groups provides some—but not all—of the nutrients you need. Foods from one group can't replace foods from another group. No one group is more important for good health—you need them all.

In Step 12 we said that, for optimum health and fitness, your body needs several essential nutrients like carbohydrates, fat and protein. Now we can see how much of these basic nutrients are contained in the six major food groups.

Fats and Sugars

Fats and refined sugars have lots of calories and little else. That's why you should eat from this food group sparingly. Remember, these fats and sugars are *added* items to other foods,

**A Serving of Fat =
0 grams carbohydrate,
0 grams protein,
5 grams fat**

57

A Serving of Sugar =
5 grams carbohydrate,
0 grams protein,
0 grams fat

especially to processed and packaged food products. Soft drinks, candy, sweetened cereals and most baked goods have lots of sugar (e.g., a can of regular soda has 9 teaspoons of sugar) and should be limited. Although no measurable standards for total sugar intake have been set by health authorities, we recommend you try to limit yourself to 8–15 teaspoons of sugar. This includes refined sugars you *add* to your food (i.e., white and brown sugar, honey and syrup) *and* sugar contained in packaged foods. Be sure to read labels for fat and sugar content, and remember, one teaspoon equals five grams of fat or sugar. (See page 367 in Charts Section for sugar servings based on body weight and activity.) ***Best Fat Choices:*** **olive and canola oil.**

58

Dairy Products

Dairy foods are the best source of calcium for strong teeth and bones. They are also rich in protein and many can be high in fat. Since dairy products come from animals, their fat content is mostly saturated. Your best bet is to choose nonfat dairy foods. If you are allergic to milk or dairy foods, a good substitute is soy-based products.

A Serving of Dairy =
12 grams carbohydrate,
8 grams protein,
0-8 grams fat

Even though cheese is a good calcium source, we do not include cheese in the dairy because the carbohydrate building block is missing. All other dairy foods contain milk sugar, which is a carbohydrate. ***Best Choices:*** **nonfat dairy products.**

Proteins

Foods in this group include all meats, eggs, cheeses, nuts and legumes. That's because these foods are all high in protein along with zinc, iron and B vitamins.

But many are high in fat also. Try to make low fat choices and remember that the fat from animal products is mostly saturated. Also, try thinking of meat and other high fat protein foods as condiments rather than the main attraction in your meals.

**A Serving of Protein =
0 grams carbohydrate,*
7 grams protein,
1–8 grams fat**

*legumes contain carbohydrates *(see page 60)*

Best Choices: **egg whites, legumes, fish, lean cuts of meat, white meat of poultry without skin and low fat cheeses.**

**A Serving of Vegetables =
5 grams carbohydrate,
2 grams protein,
trace fat**

Vegetables

Vegetables are a great source of complex carbohydrates with lots of fiber, phytochemicals (anticancer food compounds) and many of the known vitamins and minerals. As a rule, the darker or more colorful a vegetable is, the more nutrients it has. *Best Choices:* **dark, leafy greens like broccoli and spinach, carrots and tomatoes.**

59

Fruits

Fruits are another great source of complex carbohydrates with lots of fiber, phytochemicals, vitamins and some minerals. Dried fruits like prunes, raisins, and apricots are rich in iron. Citrus fruits are especially high in Vitamin C. Fruits are high in natural sugar, so they should be eaten in moderation. *Best Choices:* **whole fruits and 100% fruit juice.**

**A Serving of Fruit =
10 grams carbohydrate,
trace protein,
trace fat**

A Serving of Grains/Starches = 15 grams carbohydrate, 2 grams protein, 1 gram fat

Grains and Starches

Grains and starches give you long-lasting energy and are good sources of fiber, vitamins and minerals. Foods from this group should make up the major part of your diet. Stick to the more wholesome types of food like 100% whole wheat bread and brown rice—the more wholesome they are the more nutrients they have. Try to select at least half of your grains and starches from whole-grain sources. Remember, grains and starches are not fattening by themselves (only 1 gram of fat per serving)—it's the company they keep. **Best Choices: whole grain products, starchy vegetables (corn, yams, potatoes), brown rice and oatmeal.**

60

A Serving of Legumes = 15 grams carbohydrate, 9 grams protein, 1 gram fat

Legumes

Legumes (or beans) are a food that, in a curious way, stands on its own (legs). They are the only food which has enough carbohydrates and protein to be considered in two separate food groups—grains/starches and protein. So when you are planning your daily food servings, and you choose a serving of beans, you need to count them as one serving of starch and one serving of protein. **Best Choices: all types of beans, dried peas.**

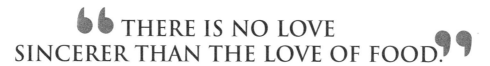

❝ THERE IS NO LOVE SINCERER THAN THE LOVE OF FOOD.❞

–George Bernard Shaw

The Food Pyramid provides a helpful way to plan your daily menus. It provides for a diet of mostly complex carbohydrates, moderate amounts of protein, small amounts of fat and sweets, and lots of fiber, vitamins and minerals. In terms of the foods to eat, it's really quite simple:

1. **Eat mostly wholesome grains and starches, legumes and vegetables.**

2. **Eat moderate amounts of fruits.**

3. **Eat small amounts of dairy, meat, eggs, cheese and nuts.**

4. **Eat fats and sugars sparingly.**

61

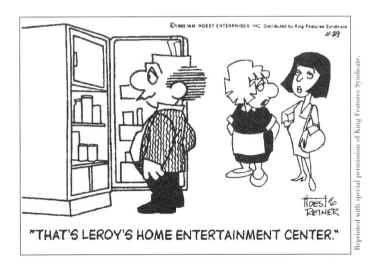

"THAT'S LEROY'S HOME ENTERTAINMENT CENTER."

STEP 14 — **Where Fat Hangs Out in the Food Pyramid**

The tippy top of the Pyramid is full of the pure fat which we *add* to our foods. But fat occurs naturally in other food groups as well, and it's important to know where. And guess what? It's concentrated in the top third of the Pyramid.

Knowing where the fat is can help you make smarter choices. When choosing your dairy or protein, you could have skim milk with zero fat or whole milk with 8 grams of fat per serving. You could have beans or egg whites with 1 gram of fat, chicken or fish with 3 grams, or sausage with 8 grams of fat per serving.

The bottom two-thirds of the Pyramid (from which we should eat the most) contain very little fat. Fruits and vegetables are living plant foods, so they need a little fat to grow but a serving of these has just a trace of fat. Grains and starches have just 1 gram of fat per serving. These foods are *not* fattening.

The chart and pyramid below illustrate the natural fat content of the different food groups in the Food Pyramid.

Food Group	Fat Content
Fats	5 grams
Sugars	0 grams
Nonfat Dairy	0 grams
Low Fat Dairy	5 grams*
Whole Dairy	8 grams*
Low Fat Protein (Legumes)	1 gram
Medium Fat Protein	3-5 grams
High Fat Protein	8 grams*
Vegetables	Trace
Fruits	Trace
Grains and Starches (Legumes)	1 gram

*A Note about Fatty Dairy/Protein Servings:

When planning your daily food servings, it is important to choose nonfat dairy products and low fat protein foods. If you choose a dairy food with fat (low fat or whole dairy products), or a high fat protein (whole egg, cheese, nuts or high fat meat), you need to count an extra serving of fat. So, if you choose to drink an 8-ounce glass of low fat milk, you need to count it as one dairy *and* one fat serving. If you choose to have an egg, an ounce of regular cheese or some sausage, you need to count each as one protein *and* one fat serving.

63

Fats and Sugars

5 GRAMS

0 GRAMS Nonfat	1 GRAM Low Fat
5 GRAMS Low Fat	3-5 GRAMS Medium Fat
8 GRAMS Whole	8 GRAMS High Fat

Dairy

Protein *(Meats, Eggs, Cheeses, Nuts, Legumes)*

Vegetables

TRACE TRACE

Fruits

1 GRAM

Grains and Starches
(Legumes)

A Note about Alcohol:

Alcoholic drinks are highly caloric (1 gram of alcohol equals 7 calories), and these calories offer no nutrients. Although alcohol does not contain any fat, it does interfere with your body's ability to burn fat, so we recommend that you count an alcoholic drink (1 ounce hard alcohol, 4 ounces wine, 12 ounces beer) as one of your servings of fat. All alcohol should be used in moderation.

STEP 15 — So What's a Serving Size?

The number of servings of the different food groups that you eat each day is really an individual thing and depends on how active you are, what your needs are, and whether or not you want to lose weight or just maintain your current weight. Step 18 will show you how many servings you should eat from each food group. So, the *number* of servings will be different for each person, but for planning your meals, the *size* of a serving will always be the same.

Let's take another look at the different food groups to find out what a serving size actually is. Here is a serving size guide for each food group, along with certain exceptions to the rule.

FOOD GROUP	SERVING SIZE GUIDE	EXCEPTIONS
Fat	1 teaspoon	Low fat dressings and mayonnaise *(1 tablespoon)*
Sugar	1 teaspoon	
Dairy	1 cup	Evaporated skim milk *(½ cup)* and nonfat frozen yogurt or ice cream *(½ cup)*
Protein	1 ounce *(Three ounces would be appropriate for a small chicken breast, piece of fish or a hamburger, and would equal 3 protein servings.)*	Egg whites *(2)* Parmesan cheese *(2 Tbsp.)* Canned tuna (in water) *(2 ounces)*
Vegetable	½ cup	Peas *(¼ cup)* and salad greens *(1 cup)*
Fruit	1 medium piece of fruit *(e.g., apple, orange, peach)* or ½ cup juice or fruit *(melons, berries)*	Grapefruit and banana *(½ fruit)* and grapes *(10)* Dried fruit *(¼ cup)*
Bread	1 slice	½ Bagel or English Muffin
Cereal *(ready-to-eat)*	¾ cup	Read labels
Grains *(pasta, rice, barley, oat, rye)*	½ cup, cooked	None
Starchy Vegetables	⅓ cup, cooked	One small potato
Legumes	½ cup, cooked	None

64

PART FOUR

Food Planning

STEP 16 — How Much Fat?

Finding a Fat Target

Or, in broader terms, we can ask: how much of everything should you eat? Back in the introduction we said *learning how to prepare and eat delicious, low fat meals without depriving yourself is one of the missing links of permanent weight loss.* We say this because we know, based on our experience, that you won't stay on any weight-loss program that deprives you of adequate amounts of good-tasting food.

So what eating habits are you going to change by starting this program? Remember that fat has more than double the calories of carbohydrates and protein, so it makes sense to focus on reducing your fat intake. Yet, it is the total number of calories you eat that will determine whether you add body fat or reduce it. The bottom line is this: whether the calories are cheeseburger calories, fat-free cookie calories or broccoli calories, extra calories from any food source will be stored as fat. So while reducing fat in your diet offers the best possibility of losing weight, if you finish off entire boxes of nonfat cookies or crackers, etc., you're not going to lose weight. So, before we look at how much fat you should eat, it's also important for you to be aware of your overall eating habits.

The average American's fat intake is about 36–40% of total calories. The American Heart

Fat has more than double the calories of carbohydrates and protein, so it makes sense to focus on reducing your fat intake.

65

FAT CHANCE

Extra calories from any food source will be stored as fat.

Association recommends that our fat intake should not exceed 30% of total calories. This is not an optimum level—it is a maximum level. The optimum level, based on the recommendations of authoritative health practitioners, is 20%. In terms of achieving permanent weight loss, this is our recommendation also.

So, while moderating our eating habits in general is helpful, we'll begin this program by adopting the goal of a maximum of 20% of our total calories from fat. Let's start by looking at the chart below, which lists the recommended grams of fat for a range of body weights. Remember grams?

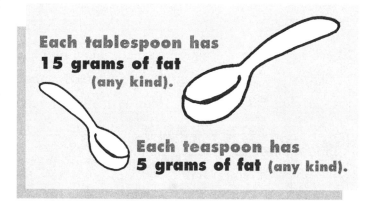

Each tablespoon has **15 grams of fat** (any kind).

Each teaspoon has **5 grams of fat** (any kind).

66

Recommended 20% Daily Fat Intake Based on Body Weight

YOUR CURRENT BODY WEIGHT IN POUNDS	RECOMMENDED GRAMS OF FAT		
	LITTLE OR NO EXERCISE	MODERATE EXERCISE	VERY ACTIVE EXERCISE
100	22	22	27
110	24	24	30
120	27	27	32
130	29	29	34
140	31	31	36
150	33	33	38
160	35	35	41
170	38	38	43
180	40	40	45
190	42	42	47
200	44	44	50

What do we mean by "Little or No Exercise," "Moderate Exercise" and "Very Active Exercise?" If you're not doing regular scheduled exercise, or if your exercise totals less than two hours per week, you're in the first category.

If you're exercising 3-4 times a week, 30-60 minutes per session, you're in the middle category. If you're exercising five or more times per week, at least 45 minutes per session, you're in the Very Active category. The exception to this is if your job requires frequent physical activity, in which case you will have to judge if you're in the Moderate or Very Active Exercise category.

**NOTE:
Though exercise is an integral part of our program, we've included the "Little or No Exercise" column for special circumstances where you are physically unable to exercise regularly, and still want to reduce your fat intake.**

67

So all you have to do is match your current body weight and level of physical activity with the recommended, daily grams of fat. If, for example, you now weigh 135 pounds and you will be starting a Moderate Exercise schedule, your daily fat target will be 30 grams.

This method of determining your daily fat intake is, of course, an approximation. But it will get you started on reducing your fat intake close to the ideal level.

Recommended Daily Fat Intake Based on Total Calories

Here's another way of figuring your ideal daily fat intake, based on total calories rather than your body weight and amount of exercise. If your ideal daily calorie total is, say, 1800, then your ideal daily fat intake should be 40 grams of fat.

YOUR IDEAL TOTAL DAILY CALORIES	RECOMMENDED FAT GRAMS/DAY BASED ON 20% OF CALORIES FROM FAT
1200	27
1400	31
1500	33
1600	36
1800	40
2000	44
2200	49
2400	53
2500	56
3000	67

Grams of Fat Per Meal

From the previous tables, you now know how many grams of fat you should be eating each day. Through the classes we teach and the many, many meals we prepare each year, we know about how much of the total daily fat intake can be allotted to each meal. Most people eat their big meal at dinner and that's why this category has the most fat. Ideally, you want to try and get most of your fat grams early in the day, so if your schedule permits you to have your big meal at lunch, then just switch the numbers accordingly. This table isn't right for everyone, of course, but it's a workable guide until you determine what is best for you.

68

Total Daily Fat in Grams	Breakfast	Lunch	Dinner	Snacks
27	4	7	12	4
31	5	7	14	5
33	6	8	14	5
36	7	9	15	5
40	7	10	18	5
44	8	11	20	5
49	8	11	24	6
53	9	13	25	6
56	10	14	25	7
67	13	16	28	10

(Here's a personal note from Joan: Actually, my own fat budget is different. I try to eat a fat-free breakfast so I can have more fat with lunch and dinner. My personal allotment looks like this:)

69

Total Daily Fat in Grams	Breakfast	Lunch	Dinner	Snacks
30	1	10	14	5

From the above tables, you now know how many grams of fat you should be eating each day, and have at least a start on how many of those fat grams you'll consume for breakfast, lunch, dinner and snacks. Be sure to write down your daily fat target in grams. Paste it in a prominent place in your kitchen—somewhere where you can't miss it when you head for the refrigerator or the snack cupboard.

Daily Fat Budget

Total Daily Fat in Grams	Breakfast	Lunch	Dinner	Snacks

You've heard about taking the "fast track?" Well, limiting your daily fat intake is the fast track to permanent weight loss. It is soooooooooo much easier than continuously counting calories and other complex methods of trying to lose weight. With our program, you can basically eat whatever you want (in moderation) as long as you limit your total daily fat. And in the following steps, we'll show you how to have yummy, satisfying, nutritious meals that are low in fat and easy to prepare.

So, in terms of the food part of our program, while you're still responsible for eating a nutritious, balanced diet, your focus will be on tracking your total daily fat intake in grams. And, as long as you're tracking fat, track the amount of saturated fat you eat too. It won't help you lose more weight, but it will benefit your overall health. So, since it can be done without much more effort, why not do it at the same time?

How do you track your total daily fat and saturated fat?

By now you have established your total daily fat target. Let's say it is 36 grams. Since your saturated fat target should be ⅓ of your total daily fat intake or less, your daily saturated fat target will be ⅓ of 36, or 12 grams of saturated fat.

Now you should have the two fat target figures that are right for you. Be sure to write them down—you'll be using them often.

Next you'll relate these two fat targets to food choices.

In the last step, you learned what your daily fat target, in grams, should be. In Step 8, we related fats to different kinds of foods and in Step 15, we showed you where fat hangs out in the Pyramid. Now you will be able to begin tracking your daily fat intake. You may also want to use this information to learn approximately how much fat you are currently consuming. Don't be surprised if your current fat intake is twice as much as, or more than your new fat target.

A sample worksheet for tracking fat is shown on the next page; copy it or use one of your own design.

If you're new to working with grams of fat in foods,

Track your daily fat intake by counting fat grams.

70

it's helpful to use one of the little handbooks that list the grams of fat in many kinds of foods. These are available in most bookstores.

Total Daily Fat Target: ▢
Daily Saturated Fat Target: ▢

Current Fat Consumption

BREAKFAST	ALL FAT IN GRAMS	SATURATED FAT IN GRAMS
LUNCH		
DINNER		
SNACKS		
	TOTAL DAY'S ALL FAT IN GRAMS	TOTAL DAY'S SATURATED FAT IN GRAMS

BREAKFAST	ALL FAT IN GRAMS	SATURATED FAT IN GRAMS
LUNCH		
DINNER		
SNACKS		
	TOTAL DAY'S ALL FAT IN GRAMS	TOTAL DAY'S SATURATED FAT IN GRAMS

71

STEP 18 — How Much Should You Eat?

By now you have a pretty clear idea of how much fat you should eat. Here we move on to asking how much, overall, you should eat. At this point, weight-loss programs typically have you starting to count calories. But with the power of the Food Pyramid, that isn't necessary. Instead, you focus on servings of food—how many servings of each kind of food should you be eating? You don't remember serving sizes? That's easy—just review Step 15.

Planning servings is a lot simpler than tracking calories, plus when you follow the Food Pyramid you know you're giving your body the good nutrition it needs and deserves.

> **Planning servings is a lot simpler than tracking calories.**

Back in Step 2, "Let's Plug Into Energy," we said that if you take in more food energy than you expend, you'll gain weight; if you take in the same amount of food energy as you expend, you'll maintain your weight; and, if you take in less food energy than you expend, you'll lose weight. Your body may resist weight changes (remember the *set point* from Step 3?) for a while, but the basic idea of energy in and energy out is valid.

So, you can theoretically lose weight by cutting back on food or increasing exercise, or both. The choice is yours. However, we have found that, for most people, the most effective way to lose weight *permanently* is to *modestly* reduce your food energy input (mostly by reducing the amount of fat you eat) and do *moderate to hard* exercise *regularly*.

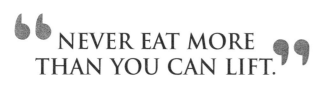

" NEVER EAT MORE THAN YOU CAN LIFT. "

–*Miss Piggy*

The following tables reflect this recommendation: a modest reduction in food intake and a moderate exercise program. They show the number of recommended servings of each food group you should eat for your body weight. The

72

top table is for losing weight and the bottom table is for maintaining the same weight—no loss or gain.

For those of you who are involved in more vigorous exercise programs, we have provided additional information on food servings in the Appendix.

RECOMMENDED DAILY FOOD GROUP SERVINGS FOR WEIGHT LOSS, BASED ON BODY WEIGHT®*

	100–120	120–140	140–160	160–180	180–200
Fat	1–2	2	2	2–3	3
Dairy	2	2	2	2	2–3
Protein	3	3–4	4–5	5–6	5–6
Vegetable	4	4–5	5	5	5–6
Fruit	3	3	3–4	4	4
Grain/Starch	5–7	7–9	9–10	10–12	12

RECOMMENDED DAILY FOOD GROUP SERVINGS FOR WEIGHT MAINTENANCE, BASED ON BODY WEIGHT®*

	100–120	120–140	140–160	160–180	180–200
Fat	2	2–3	3	3	3–4
Dairy	2	2–3	3	3	3–4
Protein	4–6	6	6–8	6–8	8
Vegetable	5–6	6	6	6	6
Fruit	4	4	4	4–5	5
Grain/Starch	9–10	10–11	11–12	12–14	14–15

73

At this point, you may want to jot down the number of servings from each food group for your body weight. The numbers may change based on your individual metabolism, lifestyle, etc., but it will help get you thinking about the kinds and amounts of food you should be eating.

---

*These numbers differ from those given by the U.S. Department of Agriculture. The USDA's numbers are lower and do not account for physical activity.

STEP 19 — **Pyramid Tracking**

In this book we have shown you a number of ways to keep track of what you're eating. Here's another. From a previous step, you've gotten a good idea of serving sizes. Being familiar with serving sizes can be very helpful, especially when that knowledge is combined with the Food Pyramid.

Remember the basic food groups of the Pyramid? Here's a reminder in this drawing:

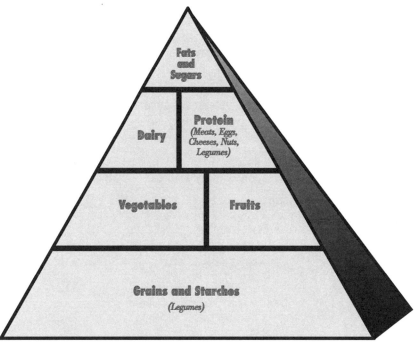

In the next drawing we show the recommended number of daily servings from each food group. In this example, the number of servings shown is for someone about 150 pounds, moderately active, who wants to lose weight. In Step 45, we will show various pyramid tracking logs based on weight and recommended food servings. So, in this example, you would be limited to 2 servings of fats, 2 dairy servings, 4 protein servings, 5 vegetable servings, 4 fruit servings and 9 grain or starch servings.

Notice that in this drawing, each food group has the number of individual sections that corresponds to the number of servings. For example, the dairy group has 2 sections, the fruit group 4 sections and so on. If you use this method for tracking your daily food intake, you'll shade in one of these sections after eating one serving from that food group.

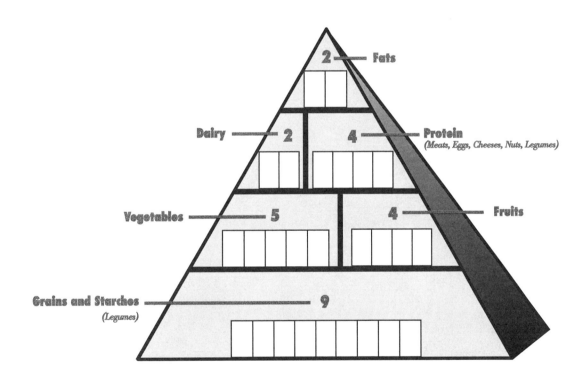

75

Next, we show a typical daily menu and how the sections of the Pyramid would be filled in to indicate what you've eaten.

On the next page is an example of Pyramid Tracking for a 150-pound person who exercises moderately, and wants to lose weight.

MEAL	FOOD GROUP SERVINGS	PYRAMID TRACKING
Breakfast: 1½ cups Wheat Chex with 1 cup skim milk and 1 banana	2 grain/starch, 1 dairy, 2 fruit	
Midmorning snack: ½ bagel with 2 tsp. peanut butter, 1 cup orange juice	1 grain/starch, 1 fat, 2 fruit	
Lunch: Bean burrito with 1 oz. low fat cheese, salad with 1 tsp. low fat dressing	2 grain/starch, 2 protein, 1 fat, 2 veggies	
Afternoon snack: 10 pretzels	1 grain/starch	
Dinner: 2 oz. chicken with 1½ cups stir-fried veggies over 1½ cups rice, with fat-free teriyaki sauce	2 protein, 3 veggies, 3 grain/starch	
Dessert: ½ cup nonfat frozen yogurt	1 dairy	

76

What about Combination Foods?

How do pizza, burritos or lasagna fit in with the food groups? It's quite simple. All you have to do is think of the different ingredients that make up these combination foods. Single items of any food group (cheese, pasta, tomato sauce), can be mixed together to form a combination food. When figuring your food servings for the day, you just break down the combo food into its various food groups. Let's take a burrito, for an example. A tasty burrito can be made with a tortilla, beans, low fat cheese and salsa or green chilies.

DISASSEMBLING A BURRITO

1 tortilla	=	1 starch
½ cup beans	=	1 starch and 1 protein
1 oz. low fat cheese	=	1 protein
¼ cup salsa or chilies	=	½ veggie
One burrito	=	**2 starches, 2 proteins and ½ veggie**

As you become more familiar with the Pyramid and its food groups, you'll find that combo foods like sandwiches or casseroles can fit into your daily food servings with just a little bit of disassembling.

The table on pages 29–31 (Step 7), showing the fat content of various foods, is divided into the six major food groups. Foods in each group are listed along with their appropriate portion size. Use this table as a guide to help you determine food servings and become more familiar with pyramid tracking. We placed high fat foods like avocados, seeds and peanut butter in the Fat Food Group because of their fat content.

When you are pyramid tracking, be sure to count an extra serving of fat for *each* serving of low fat milk, regular cheese, eggs and high fat meat you choose to eat. Count each serving of legumes as one grain/starch *and* one protein. And remember to count any alcoholic drink (1 ounce hard alcohol, 4 ounces wine, 12 ounces beer) as one serving of fat.

77

STEP 20 — **Meat Plays a Supporting Role**

It was a hit in the '50s, '60s, '70s and even in the '80s. In fact, it is still popular in our nation's midsection. Meat has played center stage for a century or more, where it has been the main attraction on dinner plates across the country.

Yet, times are changing. The relationship between meat and higher incidences of colon cancer and heart disease are booing meat off center stage. Does this mean it should be banned completely from our plates? No, because meat is an extremely good source of protein, B vitamins, zinc and iron. Yet, it's also rich in unwanted saturated fat and cholesterol. So the trick is to balance meat with other foods that are low in fat, such as veggies, fruits, beans, breads and grains.

> **Start thinking of meat as a condiment or side dish, instead of the main attraction.**

Meat performs best in a supporting role. Start thinking of it as a condiment or side dish, instead of as the main attraction. Here are a few suggestions:

- Think of a deck of playing cards as about the right size for a single serving of meat. This size is about a 3-ounce serving.
- When you stir-fry, cut meat into thin strips to go alongside your veggies.
- When making a spaghetti meat sauce, use extra lean meat (ground round) and use only ½ the amount the recipe calls for. If you prefer the taste of sausage, use only enough to get the flavor and combine it with lean ground round.
- To replace ground meat in spaghetti sauce or chili, try adding textured vegetable protein (found at your local health food store) or substitute ground mushrooms as a thickener.
- Replace high fat meats, such as pepperoni, sausage, bacon, hot dogs and lunch meats with lean or low fat choices of poultry, beef or pork.
- Trim off any fat on solid cuts of meat and avoid eating the skin (which has a very high fat content).
- Serve little chunks of steak instead of a 12-ouncer.

- When preparing shish kebabs, skewer 3 cubes of meat with your veggies instead of 6 cubes.
- Add *small* chunks of meat to noodle and rice dishes.
- Large Portobello mushrooms are a great substitute for steak; season them with herbs and grill, sauté or barbeque them.
- Avoid restaurants where meat is the specialty, such as barbequed rib places, hamburger joints and steak houses.

❝ WE USED TO SAY, 'WHAT'S COOKING?' WHEN WE CAME HOME FROM WORK. NOW IT'S, 'WHAT'S THAWING?' ❞

–Jacob Brande

Here is an added incentive to use meat in a supporting role: Around the world, several ethnic groups are known to live longer and be healthier than "normal." The best known of these groups is the Hunza people, who live in the Himalayas between India and Pakistan. All of these long-living groups share several things in common. We list them here:

- A strong spiritual life.
- Very close families.
- Clean air and water.
- Diet consists primarily of vegetables, grains, fruits and small amounts of meat.
- Rigorous daily exercise (such as daily trekking through mountains to and from crop fields).
- No one retires or becomes sedentary—as long as they live.

Of course, no one can say for sure which of these elements contributes most to the extraordinary vigor and longevity of these people, but we do know that, for ourselves, we'll be healthier, more trim and fit, we'll probably live longer—and we'll even save money—by getting into the new meat habit.

It's tasty, it's chewy, it's great—*on the side.*

79

STEP 21 — **Menu Planning and Shopping**

Often, we don't allow enough time for meal preparation, or we don't have the right ingredients available at home—there are dozens of reasons why we don't prepare healthy, satisfying, low fat meals. What almost all of the reasons have in common is lack of planning. Meal planning is one of the keys to eating right, and eating right is a necessary requirement for permanent weight loss.

Once again, it's a matter of changing your habits. When you begin planning your weekly meals, we think you'll find this new habit very helpful. And if the rest of your family joins in, the process is not only productive—it's fun.

Help with Meal Planning

- Keep a well-stocked pantry and take the time to create your own personal grocery list of "essentials" that you always want to have on hand. Include every item that you buy at the store—from foods to paper goods to cleaning supplies. Then, make lots of copies so that you can start with a clean list every week. Keep your grocery list on the refrigerator or in a designated spot so that family members can check items that you are out of or need. Once your list is made up anyone can go to the store and get the needed supplies. Appendix A shows a sample list of essential items; you can use it as a starting point and modify it to suit your own needs.

Plan two Veggie Nights a week!

- Set up a card file with a complete meal on each card. Ask family members to help by reminding you of all of their favorite dishes, or have them fill out a card or two. On each card, list the ingredients required for that meal.
- Plan two nights of each week as "Veggie Nights" to lower the amount of saturated fat consumed by your family. Be sure to space them out, leaving two or three days between each "Veggie Night." Instead of using meat, prepare:

80

Soups
Salads
Potatoes
Veggie stir-fry
Veggie pizza (no cheese)
Beans
Stuffed veggies
Casseroles
Grilled veggies
(See Step 25 — "Veggie Power," for lots more ideas)

- To make life easier, bring home a prepared dinner once a week, such as pizza, Japanese, Chinese or Mexican. Scout out the restaurants in your area that offer take-out meals that complement your meal planning. Then you can phone or fax your order half an hour or so before you head for home and pick it up on the way—or have another family member pick it up. This gives you at least one evening a week with more time and less cleanup. Expensive? With a bit of careful selection, you'll find some good take-out meals that cost about the same as, or only a little more, than it would cost you to make them at home. Plus, you can use the extra time for planning the weekly menu, which will save you both time and money each week.

- Set aside one day a week for planning the weekly menu. If you have a card file, you can pull out a number of cards for the entire week and list all the ingredients you'll need from them. Also, plan the day you will do the weekly shopping. Yes, it takes a bit of time to do this, but you'll find it saves you much more time because you won't have to decide what to make each day and whether or not you have all the ingredients on hand. (See the Sample Plan for a Week, which follows in this step.)

81

- On each card of your card file, list the name of the family member who requested that meal. Then, when it's time to prepare those meals, remind family members that you're making one of their favorite meals and get them to help you with it.
- Get ideas for new meals from restaurants, friends, cookbooks, magazines, etc. Have space near your "essentials" list where family members can jot down their suggestions for meals. Try to get the whole family involved.

Mix and Match

Here are some basic foods to help you start planning the components of your meals.

GRAINS/STARCHES	VEGGIES	PROTEINS
Bread	Green veggies	Poultry
Pasta	Yellow veggies	Fish
Rice	Salad greens	Red meat
Potatoes	Underground veggies	Pork tenderloin
Tortillas	Carrots	Low Fat Cheese
Cornbread	Tomato Sauce or Salsa	Beans
Bulgur/Barley	Eggplant	Eggs
Pizza Crust	Mushrooms	Nuts
Polenta	Onions, Garlic, Parsley	Soy Protein (Tofu)

How much of each category should you plan to use? The Food Pyramid tells us that the largest number of servings should be from grains and starches, followed by vegetables and fruits and protein, and then dairy and fat. Putting it another way, the proportion of daily servings from each food group is represented by the blocks shown below. So, for the above Mix and Match foods, plan on about twice as many servings of grains and starches as veggies and protein.

82

Relative Number of Daily Servings from Each Food Group

Sample Meal Plans

SAMPLE MEAL PLAN FOR A DAY

(This meal plan is appropriate for someone about 150 lbs., moderately active, who wants to lose weight.)

Meal	Food	Food Group Servings
Breakfast	1½ cups ready-to-eat cereal	2 starches
	1 cup skim milk	1 dairy
	½ banana	1 fruit
Midmorning snack	1 apple	1 fruit
Lunch	Salad with 1 Tbsp. low fat dressing	2 veggies, 1 fat
	Bean burrito w/1 oz. low fat cheese	2 proteins, 2 starches
Midafternoon snack	4 graham crackers (2 lg. rectangles)	1 starch
	1 cup orange juice	2 fruits
Dinner	Spaghetti and meatballs (1½ cups pasta w/2 oz. lean meat, ½ cup sauce)	4 starches
		2 proteins
	1 pc. garlic bread w/1 tsp. butter,	1 fat
	1 cup steamed veggies	3 veggies
Dessert	½ cup nonfat yogurt	1 dairy

83

SAMPLE MEAL PLAN FOR A WEEK OF DINNERS

Day	Recipe Idea	Grain/Starch	Veggie	Protein
Monday	Linguini with clams	Pasta	Yellow veggies	Clams
Tuesday	Bean burritos	Corn tortillas, Rice	Salsa, Salad	(Veggie Night) Beans
Wednesday	Veggie pizza	Pizza crust	Various veggies, Tomato sauce	Low Fat Cheese
Thursday	Chicken sauté w/roasted potatoes	Potatoes	Mushrooms, Spinach	Chicken
Friday	Grilled fish	Rice	Green veggies	Fish
Saturday	Pasta primavera	Pasta	Various veggies	(Veggie Night)
Sunday	Flank steak w/garlic mashed potatoes	Potatoes	Artichokes	Red meat

Try planning menus for several weeks. Work with the seasons, using fresh produce that becomes available at different times of the year.

Here's a time-saver. Cook twice the amount of baked potatoes, rice or pasta you need and use it in another form the next day. Have fun with your grains and starches. When planning meals for the week, try planning a:

- Pasta night
- Baked potato night
- Rice night
- Tortilla night
- Polenta night
- French fry night
- Mashed potato night

A Shopping Tip

One hundred years ago there were no grocery stores as we know them: there were only markets that sold fresh produce, meats and fish, fresh bakery goods,

84

> **❝ I ALWAYS PLAN DINNER FIRST THING IN THE MORNING. THAT'S THE ONLY WAY I CAN GET THROUGH THE DAY, HAVING A SPECIFIC MEAL TO LOOK FORWARD TO AT NIGHT. ❞**
>
> *—Alan King*

and usually a good assortment of dried staples, such as flour, beans, corn and rice. Very few grocery products were packaged or had anything added to them—perhaps salt to help preserve the fish. As a consequence, people ate real food . . . what we call *Pyramid Food.* Then, during World War I, the British set up supply stations to get food to their soldiers, and they began to package food and store it. Of course, sitting there in the boxes, it gradually became too hard or too soft or lost its natural color, so additives were invented to maintain its natural appearance.

This trend toward packaged, stabilized, colorized, flavorized food expanded dramatically, especially in the U.S., and today most of the food that is sold is of this kind.

85

Walk around a supermarket and look. Three-quarters of all the food displayed is processed. Interestingly enough, in almost every supermarket the processed foods are displayed in the *center* of the store. Walk around the periphery and you see fresh baked goods, fresh dairy products, fresh meat, and fresh produce. So here's a walking guide for supermarkets—stick to the outside aisles and let the majority of the foods you buy be real foods . . . fresh foods . . . Pyramid Foods.

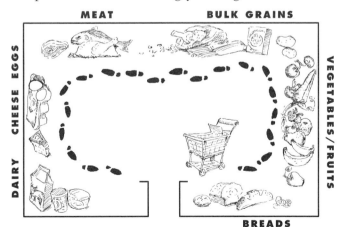

Do most of your shopping on the outside aisles of your supermarket—that's where the real food is!

Plan for a Week of Dinners

Day	Recipe Idea	Grain/Starch	Veggie	Protein
Monday				
Tuesday				
Wednesday				
Thursday				
Friday				
Saturday				
Sunday				

86

STEP 22 — **What about Doughnuts?**

Y ou may have noticed that certain foods—certain favorite foods, are not even mentioned in the Food Pyramid. That's because they fall under the fat and sugar group and you know you should eat sparingly from this group. But sometimes, you just gotta have a doughnut! So what can you do?

We think it's important that, if you choose a certain high fat food, you know just how much fat you are eating and how this amount fits in with your daily fat target. So, we have provided a list of foods outside of the Pyramid and given you their fat content.

FATTY FOOD	FAT GRAMS	REMAINING FAT GRAMS FOR THE DAY (Based on a 33 gram fat target)
Bread Pudding (1 cup)	16	17
Brownie (2" by 2")	7	26
Butterfinger (2 oz.)	11	22
Cake, from mix ($1/_{12}$ slice)	11	22
New York Cheesecake (⅛ slice)	14	19
Chicken Nuggets (6)	18	15
Chocolate Chip Cookie (homemade)	4	29
Chocolate Chips (handful)	12	21
Cinnamon Bun (1)	9	24
Croissant (1)	19	14
Danish Pastry (1)	9	24
Doughnut (Glazed, raised)	12	21
Éclair (1)	13	20
Egg McMuffin (1)	16	17
Eggnog (1 cup)	19	14
Fettucine Alfredo (1 cup)	20	13
French Fries (regular size)	12	21

87

Fatty Food	Fat Grams	Remaining Fat Grams for the Day (Based on a 33 gram fat target)
Fudge (1 oz.)	4	29
Ice Cream (Vanilla, ½ cup)	8	25
Hot Dog (1)	14	19
Kit Kat Bar (1.5 oz.)	12	21
Milk Chocolate Bar (1 oz.)	9	24
Nachos (1 serving)	35	-2
Oreos (3)	6	27
Peanut Butter Cups (2)	17	16
Peanut M&M's (handful)	12	21
Pie (Apple, ⅛ slice)	11	22
Pie à la Mode	17	16
Potato Chips (1 oz.)	10	23
Snickers Bar (2 oz.)	14	19
Sundae (½ cup)	10	23
Twinkie (1)	5	28

You can see that just a tiny bit of these foods can blow your fat budget. If you choose to eat from outside the Food Pyramid, be prepared to eat low fat and nonfat foods the rest of day.

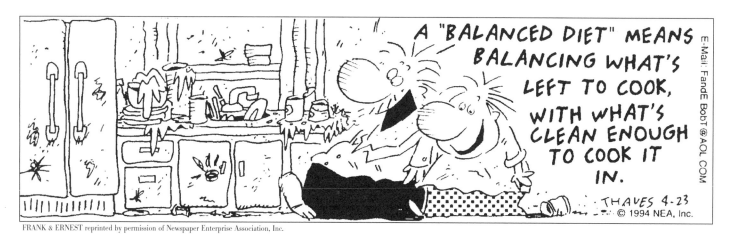

FRANK & ERNEST reprinted by permission of Newspaper Enterprise Association, Inc.

PART FIVE

Delicious Low Fat Cooking Techniques

STEP 23 — Using Fat in Cooking and Baking

We would like you to learn concepts rather than focus on recipes. We'll present recipes, in all categories from soups to desserts, but these recipes are only aids to learning low fat cooking methods. You'll be using your own recipes, too—your tried-and-true recipes can be creatively altered to lower their fat content and still taste good!

Our emphasis on low fat eating will be more on cooking creatively than on dieting, and more on pleasure than denial. It will be a fun learning experience. There is more to healthy eating than just nutrition

> **KISSING DON'T LAST; COOKERY DO.**
> —*George Meredith*

89

and cooking techniques—it's inviting friends and family to enjoy good food. It's like directing a beautiful movie scene. The lights are dimmed, the fireplace is blazing, the candles are lit and flowers are on the table. There is the clink of glasses with the ruby red glow of wine reflecting friendship as someone proposes a toast. It's the fellowship, warmth and conversation that gives us the feeling of well-being. It's to connect and nurture our bodies and our souls. And it's the healthy cooking that will keep us around to enjoy these precious moments.

As cooks we are used to automatically pouring oil in a pan when cooking a meal for the family. We have been told by generations before us that oil is needed to make things golden, crispy and tasty. Well, fat does improve flavor and texture, but we have found that you can still get the flavor and texture you want with less fat, and sometimes with no fat at all. So we'll describe how to cook with less fat by giving you five basic techniques. If you wish, you can use one technique for lunch and a different technique for dinner, depending on who you are cooking for, the results you want and your personal daily target of fat consumption.

To see how the following techniques can change the amount of fat you would use in a recipe, we will first show you an example of how to count your fat in a recipe and then compare the different methods with this recipe.

Example of Counting Fats in a Recipe

CHICKEN SAUTÉ FOR SIX PEOPLE

Ingredients	Fat Grams
(main dish)	
2 tablespoons sesame, olive or canola oil	30
4 chicken breast halves (trim all fat), 22 ounces	22
1 cup bean sprouts	0
½ cup red bell pepper	0
4 green onions	0
1 cup broccoli	0
1 tablespoon fresh ginger	0
(sauce)	
1 tablespoon cornstarch	0
½ cup marsala wine	0
½ cup defatted chicken broth	0
¼ cup lite soy sauce	0
total fat grams:	52

When we divide the 52 grams of fat by six servings, it comes out to 8.6 grams of fat per person, which will fit nicely into anyone's daily fat budget.

90

If you use beef or pork in this recipe, it will increase the grams of fat per serving. Note the differences in the following:

• Skinless chicken has 1 gram of fat per ounce. Multiply by 22 ounces of meat in the recipe = 22 grams of fat. Add this to the 30 grams from the 2 Tbsp. of oil, for a total of 52 grams of fat in the recipe, which is *8.6 grams of fat per serving*.

• Lean beef and pork have 3 grams of fat per ounce. Multiply by 22 ounces of meat in the recipe = 66 grams of fat. Add this to the 30 grams from the 2 Tbsp. of oil, for a total of 96 grams of fat in the recipe, which is *16 grams of fat per serving*.

This recipe could work as a lunch dish or dinner dish over rice cooked in broth (no fat added), or over fettucine (no fat added). If we used chicken as the meat ingredient, and our allotment of fat for dinner was, say, 15 grams, we would have enough fat grams left for a nice side dish or two. We might, for example, sauté bok choy, spinach or chard as a side dish along with a nonfat sorbet for dessert—and still come out below our fat budget for dinner.

Now, we have the five techniques of cooking with less fat.

The Five Basic Techniques

1. **Pouring a calculated amount of oil into a pan.**

2. **Spraying the pan with an aerosol or pump nonstick cooking spray.**

3. **Putting oil on a paper towel to coat the pan.**

4. **Using broth, wine, or other nonfat liquids to coat the pan.**

5. **Using nothing in the pan (tricky, but can be done with the proper pan).**

91

Each tablespoon has 15 grams of fat (any kind).

Each teaspoon has 5 grams of fat (any kind).

1. Pouring a Calculated Amount of Oil into a Pan

How much oil do we pour into a pan? For most of us, we pour what looks like the right amount, just as we have been doing for years. We do this without much thought to how many grams of fat we are adding. But remember, all fats, oils or butter are 5 grams of fat per teaspoon and 15 grams of fat per tablespoon.

How much fat is necessary to get the good results you want? Based on considerable testing, what we practice and recommend is to use 5 grams of fat per serving.

Using the Chicken Sauté for six people example, we'll use 5 grams of fat, which multiplied by 6 people equals 30 grams of fat. This is the equivalent of 2 tablespoons, and is the amount we'll add to the pan. *So, with the first method we are adding 30 grams of fat.*

We use 5 grams of fat per serving.

2. Using an Aerosol or Pump Nonstick Cooking Spray

We are fortunate that most oils now come in a nonstick pump or aerosol spray. These sprays include canola oil, vegetable oil and olive oil. We recommend you keep one of each handy at your stove. Read the directions carefully on each can. Some contain alcohol, so you don't spray it on a hot pan or near an open flame— or you could cause a fire. Shake the can and hold it upright, approximately 12" from the pan, spraying for about 2½ seconds to coat the pan surface. This should be repeated 2 to 3 times when moving potatoes and vegetables in the pan in order to brown them on all sides.

92

Aerosol cooking sprays are handy for:
- Sautéing meats and vegetables.
- Frying or browning potatoes, meats and eggs.
- Coating potatoes and vegetables when roasting in an oven.
- Grilling sandwiches.
- Using as the oil portion for salad dressings.

Mazola No Stick Corn Oil Cooking Spray has about ¾ of a gram of fat for each 2¾ seconds of spray. Spraying this product 8–16 times gives you 6–12 grams of fat for the sautéed chicken recipe. *Canola Harvest Nonstick Spray* is essentially fat-free per spray, and 8–16 sprayings of this gives you 3¼–6½ grams of fat per recipe. These examples are given only to make you aware that each cooking spray has different amounts of oil and ingredients. Using aerosol sprays for the sautéed chicken recipe *would add between 3¼–12 grams of fat, depending on which brand of spray you choose.*

93

3. Using a Paper Towel with Oil

This method of coating the pan gives you very little fat, but needs to be done with a good pan. You will end up with 3–5 grams per application depending on the paper towel absorption. This technique makes it more difficult to precisely figure fat grams, but it is very useful for those who prefer not to use aerosol nonstick cooking spray.

Using the same Chicken Sauté recipe for six persons, before sautéing, you would pour a teaspoon of oil into your pan. Using a paper towel you would coat your pan and then make sure you stir your ingredients well. Therefore, *with this technique, you would use 3–5 grams of fat compared to 30 grams of fat if you were to pour 2 tablespoons of oil into the pan.*

4. Using Broth, Wine or Other Nonfat Liquid to Coat Your Pan

When you use chicken or beef broth, always take all the fat off the top of the broth with a spoon. Incidentally, the fat in these broths is a great example of how fat looks different depending on how saturated it is. Compare the fat on the top of a beef broth can to the fat on the top of a chicken broth can. The beef fat consists of hard, white curds (more saturated) while the chicken fat is soft, like an oil slick on water (less saturated).

If you are a purist and want no fat at all from the broth, put it in the refrigerator to get a better separation of the fat from the broth, or buy brands that say "nonfat." Vegetable broth and wine have no fat and can be used as-is.

Refrigerate broth to solidify any fat.

Red and white wine can be used like a broth. When you get it hot in your sauté pan, the alcohol will burn off and you will be left with the rich and gentle flavor of wine.

It's a bit harder to judge the amount of broth or wine to use with a dish. It will depend on the size of your pan and the amount of food you want to sauté. We suggest starting with ¼ cup to ⅓ cup broth or wine in a 10" or 12" pan. Put your broth in the pan and then turn up the heat to medium-high or high. You can sauté one vegetable at a time or two or three at a time, depending on ingredient amounts. You don't want to boil or steam the ingredients, you want to sauté them. That means you keep adding just enough broth or wine to the pan so foods don't stick or burn, but not so much that you are steaming or boiling them. By doing this, you should be able to get a nice, glazed brown look.

The advantage of this method is you're not adding any fat, so you can keep adding broth/wine in abundance.

We like to use a ⅔ broth, ⅓ wine mixture to sauté or stir-fry.

94

This is an excellent method to prepare a typical stir-fry or sauté, as the broth and wine greatly enhance the flavor of the dish. We like to use a ⅔ broth, ⅓ wine mixture to sauté or stir-fry.

5. Dry-Pan Cooking

Low fat and nonfat cooking sprays are now readily available. But there is actually a small amount of fat in the "nonfat" sprays—the amount is small enough so that they can be legally called "nonfat." So the only time to consider dry-pan cooking is when you can't use a wine, broth or other nonfat liquid, and you must restrict fat to the absolutely smallest possible amount. Dry-pan cooking is tricky and must be done with a very good pan. What's a very good pan? As a starter, we never recommend inexpensive, Teflon-coated pans. The Teflon can't take the repeated use of high heat, and it starts breaking up. The best pans are very hard, very smooth, thick-walled stainless steel (thin-walled stainless steel pans don't hold enough heat and don't distribute it evenly). Some of the pans that are on the market now are 75 percent harder than the pans of a few years ago. One brand name in this new generation of pans is *Analon*. We have also found some of the older pans like *Commercial Cookware* and *Calphalon* can be used with this technique.

95

Certain kinds of foods are easier to dry-sauté than others. Vegetables are easiest because of their high moisture content, and the hardest are probably eggs and potatoes. What you are doing with the dry-pan technique is using the moisture in the ingredients to get the sauté effect. The trick with this technique is to allow the ingredients to remain in one place just long enough to brown—and the time between brown and burnt is short. Then they must be immediately stirred so all the food surfaces come in contact with the pan.

This technique is comparable to the broth/wine technique because there are no fats added.

To summarize the above methods:

Cooking Technique	Ways You Can Use this Technique	Amount of Fat Added, in Grams per Person (Chicken Sauté Recipe)
Spooning fat into the pan	Grilling, sautéing, baking, frying	5
Using an aerosol or pump cooking spray	Grilling, sautéing, baking, frying	0–3
Putting oil on a paper towel to coat the pan	Grilling, sautéing, baking, frying	0–2
Using broth or wine to coat the pan	Sautéing, baking, steaming	0
Using a dry pan (must be proper pan)	Sautéing	0

Baking

The smell of homemade baked goods fills a house with warmth and can bring anyone into the kitchen to find out "What's bakin'?" But baking is different from cooking in a fundamental way, and people often classify themselves as either a cook or a baker. Part of the reason for this is that with cooking you can experiment more with ingredients and with baking you have to be more exact. Cooking has been compared to art, while baking is more like a science. Rarely does a person feel competent at both. But we're here to tell you that you can be successful at *taking the fat out* whether it's cooking or baking.

So far we've given you techniques and substitutions to lower the fat in cooking. Now we'll give you some ideas for doing the same in baking.

Don't try to eliminate all of the fat from a cake or other baked goods—you need to have a little.

Fats like butter, shortening, oil and cream play an important role in baking. They add moisture and consistency to a cake, tenderness to a batter, flakiness to a crust. The whipping of sugars and fats in a recipe creates air pockets that play a significant role in the texture and taste of the finished baked item.

Some recipes have always had too much fat, so taking a little out won't change the texture very much. Don't try to eliminate all of the fat from a cake or other baked goods, though—you need to have a little. But when you do take half or more of the fat out, you need some guidelines to help you be successful.

Substitutions to Lower the Fat in Baking

• Whip sugars with egg or egg substitute in place of butter or shortening
Even a real egg has less fat than if you use butter or shortening. You can create the same effect of air pockets in the batter while dramatically reducing the fat content.

• Use fruit or sweet vegetable purées in place of fats
Fats in a baking recipe also serve as moisteners. An effective substitution is to use a fruit butter or sweet vegetable purée to replace half or more of the fat ingredients. Some examples of purées are puréed bananas, apples, prunes, pears, pumpkins, sweet potatoes and carrots. So, if your baking recipe calls for 8 ounces of butter, try 4 ounces of butter and 4 ounces of prune purée. A fresh fruit purée is also a great substitute for whipped cream—serve baked desserts topped with a fresh fruit sauce or on a bed of puréed raspberries instead of with cream.

• Add liquid sweeteners for moisture
Yet another technique to add back moisture that is taken away when fat is reduced is to add a liquid sweetener such as molasses, maple syrup or corn syrup (take it easy with these—they don't have fat but they do have calories). We often use a natural sweetener, like honey, instead of white sugar in our recipes. If you do this, the correct substitution is ¾ cup liquid sweetener for every 1 cup of dry refined sugar.

97

- **Substitution in a pie crust**

Use low fat cottage cheese to replace half of the shortening or butter, and decrease the liquid content slightly.

- **Substitution for crème fraîche**

Traditionally, this is a very heavy cream with 35% butterfat! Try making it with a carton of nonfat ricotta cheese, a dash of vanilla and 6 tablespoons of nonfat vanilla yogurt. Whip in a blender for 5 minutes and refrigerate overnight for best results.

- **Substitution for eggs in baking**

For 2 whole eggs, substitute 1 whole egg plus 2 egg whites; or use a good egg substitute either to completely replace the eggs or in combination with 1 whole egg.

- **Substitution for cream in baking**

Good alternatives are buttermilk, yogurt cheese (see our recipe in the Sauces section), or use the crème fraîche substitution described above.

- **Substitution for cream cheese and sour cream in baking**

There are many good low fat and nonfat products now on the market. Use them!

- **Substitution for whole milk in baking**

Low fat, nonfat and evaporated skim milk work well as substitutes in most baking recipes.

- **Substitution for baker's chocolate in baking**

Try substituting Dutch process cocoa powder or regular cocoa powder. These two products are both lower in fat than baker's chocolate (bars of chocolate). When *baking powder* is present in the recipe use regular cocoa instead of Dutch process cocoa because the latter will interfere with how the dessert rises, leaving it sticky and gummy.

98

- **Substitution for chocolate chips in baking**

Use mini-chocolate chips instead of regular size ones. This way you can cut back on the amount you use and still get an even distribution of chocolate throughout the dessert.

- **Substitution for nuts in baking**

Either decrease the total amount of nuts in the recipe or replace half of the nuts with raisins, dates, figs or other dried fruit.

In general, always use the highest quality ingredients to get the best results in your baking recipes. Flavored liqueurs are a nice addition to many baking recipes as they heighten flavor and add moisture to the finished product.

There are some very good low fat baking and dessert cookbooks on the market. Look them over and find the one(s) that best suit your baking style. The key is not to be afraid to change the recipe by lowering the fat content. You may have to experiment a few times with a recipe, but after you have found the correct balance of ingredients, it will all be worth it. Then you'll be able to have your cake and eat it, too!

99

STEP 24 — The Art of Low Fat Food Substitution

Nowadays there is an array of substitutions in the supermarket that allows us more choice and flexibility in lowering the fat in recipes than ever before. This step will show you how to substitute low fat ingredients for breakfast, lunch and dinner, without depriving yourself of tasty, satisfying meals.

Let's Start with Breakfast

In the good old days, depending on your age and appetite, it was acceptable to have sugar-coated cereal, sausage and eggs, fried potatoes and French toast with lots of melted butter and syrup for breakfast—plus coffee with thick cream. Today we know better and eat differently. Breakfast is a very important meal of the day and we certainly shouldn't skip it, but we know we should keep our daily fat consumption to 20% or less of total calories. Most of us work and have little time to prepare a large breakfast while we're getting ourselves ready or getting the kids off to school. So we need a variety of nonfat or low fat breakfast choices that we can depend on.

Cereal, of course, is one of the first things that comes to mind. There is such a variety in the amount of fat in different cereals that you need to choose carefully. For instance, look at the two cereals below. The labels on the boxes read as follows:

CEREAL	SIZE	CALORIES	FAT
Crispix	1 cup	110	1
Low fat granola	⅓ cup	110	2

Notice that the figures for the low fat granola are for only ⅓ cup. If we want to compare 1 cup to 1 cup, look at the difference in the amount of fat for the same volume.

CEREAL	SIZE	CALORIES	FAT
Crispix	1 cup	110	1
Low fat granola	1 cup	330	6

Six grams of fat per cup for so-called low fat granola! That's a considerable amount of fat. In contrast, you can have up to 6 cups of Crispix for the same amount of fat.

Next, let's look at one of our favorite breakfasts. Five or six days a week we like ½ of a toasted bagel with nonfat vanilla yogurt and a sliced banana or other fresh fruit on top. A cappuccino with nonfat hot milk accompanies it. This breakfast has just a trace of fat.

For a weekend breakfast we use Krusteaz buttermilk pancake mix with nonfat yogurt, "lite" syrup, and fruit. This comes out to be about 3 grams of fat per three, 4" pancakes.

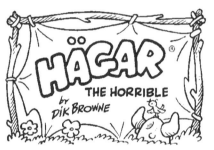
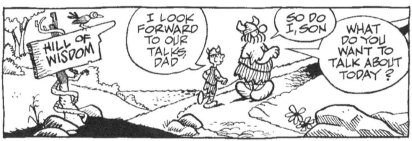

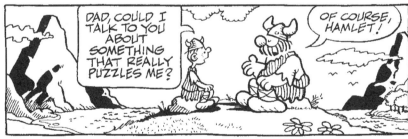
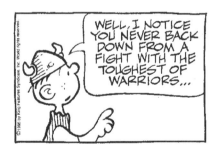

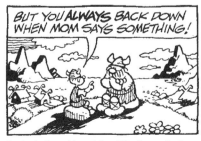
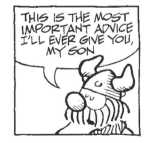
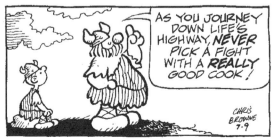

Reprinted with special permission of King Features Syndicate.

Another of our favorite weekend breakfasts is Huevos Rancheros. Here's how to prepare it:

1. Heat a flour tortilla (1 gram of fat) in a nonstick pan (a hard, stainless steel type as previously recommended).

2. Microwave some nonfat, refried beans. Use approximately 3 tablespoons per serving.

3. Spray the pan with oil (a fraction of a gram of fat) and fry 1 whole egg (6 grams of fat) and 1 egg white.

4. Place the fried egg on the tortilla and place the warm beans so they are circling the egg.

5. Place 2 teaspoons of chopped green chiles, fresh salsa and nonfat sour cream to decorate on top of and around the beans.

102

This version of Huevos Rancheros is 6 grams of fat per serving. How does that fit into your daily fat target? Let's take another look at the table that allots grams of fat for each meal. Remember, this table is just one way of allotting fat per meal—your preferences may be quite different.

Total Daily Fat in Grams	Breakfast	Lunch	Dinner	Snacks
27	4	7	12	4
31	5	7	14	5
33	6	8	14	5
36	7	9	15	5
40	7	10	18	5
44	8	11	20	5
49	8	11	24	6
53	9	13	25	6
56	10	14	25	7
67	13	16	28	10

As you can see, the 6 grams of fat for breakfast will fit most people—at least all of those whose total daily fat target is 33 grams or more. And even for those whose target is less than 33 grams of daily fat, this recipe is meant to be a once-a-week meal. The other breakfast meals during the week will probably have a lower fat content.

In addition to a delicious breakfast, this Huevos Rancheros recipe makes a nice brunch, lunch or dinner on a Sunday.

Lunch Salads

When you buy lettuce, wash it and put it in a plastic bag in the refrigerator. Salads are a good choice and if the lettuce is clean and ready to tear, you will make salads more often—because half the work is already done. So, when you buy lettuce, get into the habit of washing it and putting it in a plastic bag right after you put your groceries away. If you're not already doing it, try the following low fat substitutions in your salads.

INSTEAD OF THIS	TRY THIS
Artichoke hearts in oil	Frozen artichoke hearts or canned hearts in water
Regular oil and vinegar	Low fat or nonfat commercial dressings or our recipes
Sliced avocados	Roasted red pepper
Sliced olives	One olive sliced lengthwise
Mushrooms in oil	Fresh sliced mushrooms
Sesame seeds	Kidney beans
Almonds	Garbanzo beans
Hard-boiled whole egg	Hard-boiled egg whites
Regular mayonnaise	Lite or nonfat mayonnaise

Salad Dressings

There are some basic low fat and nonfat salad dressings in the recipe section of this book, such as Honey-Mustard, Green Goddess and Creamy Caesar. Try them and don't be afraid to adjust them to your taste. Or, use your own favorite recipes and substitute a low or nonfat product where the fat products are. Keep two of your favorite homemade dressings in the refrigerator at all times, or two commercial dressings you enjoy.

INSTEAD OF THIS	TRY THIS
Oil for dressing	Half oil and half wine
Cream	Nonfat cottage cheese blended with nonfat plain yogurt or ½ nonfat yogurt and ½ Yogurt Cheese recipe (see Dressings section in recipes)
Half & Half	½ low fat or nonfat buttermilk and ½ nonfat vanilla yogurt
Regular commercial dressings	Low or nonfat commercial dressings, and see our low fat dressings recipes

Lunch Sandwiches

Now that you know some good choices for a salad, let's add a sandwich, a taco or a pizza with it.

INSTEAD OF THIS	TRY THIS
White bread	Whole grain bread or pita bread
Mayonnaise	Lite mayonnaise or mustard, or ½ cup nonfat mayonnaise mixed with 1 Tbsp. Dijon-style mustard and 1 tsp. horseradish
Bologna slices	Lite turkey or chicken slice
Cheese slices	Lite cheese slices
Avocado slices	Fresh mushroom slices, Mezzeta's marinated red bell pepper slices or our low fat Tomacilantro Guacamole recipe

If you want a grilled sandwich, just spray your pan with an aerosol nonstick spray prior to grilling. This can add 1 gram of fat or less, depending on the spray you choose. If you mix some nonfat cottage cheese with some grated low fat cheese and green chiles, it makes a nice, moist, low fat grilled sandwich. It may sound weird, but it works!

Tacos

Mexican food doesn't have to be fattening if you know how to cook it the low fat way. We fix a Mexican lunch every few days. There is nothing like a warm tortilla with beans and chiles.

INSTEAD OF THIS	TRY THIS
Flour tortilla (6 fat grams)	Low fat flour tortilla or corn tortilla (1 fat gram each)
1 oz. cheese, shredded (8–10 fat grams)	1 oz. lite cheese shredded (4 fat grams)
Avocado 1/2 slice (8 fat grams)	Green chiles, whole or chopped (0 fat) or low fat guacamole
Beef, shredded	Lean turkey, chicken or fish, shredded
Refried beans in lard	Nonfat refried beans
Sour cream	Nonfat sour cream

Pizza

Pizza is a great food for the family, and starting with a plain Boboli (baked Italian pizza crust), you can top it with creative low fat ingredients and make it for an afterschool treat.

105

INSTEAD OF THIS	TRY THIS
High fat crust	Low fat Boboli
Cheese	Lite cheese
Olives	Grilled veggies
Pepperoni	Lite ham or Canadian bacon
Sausage	Lean chicken or turkey, lite sausage or shrimp
Tomato sauce with oil	Nonfat tomato sauce

Soups

Soups are a great filler for summer or winter, cold or hot. They can also supply you and your family with lots of delicious complex carbohydrates by using noodles and rice, and a variety of fresh vegetables.

INSTEAD OF THIS	TRY THIS
Regular chicken broth	Defatted chicken broth
8 tablespoons butter	4 tablespoons butter and 4 tablespoons white wine or Madeira, or use 8 tablespoons of Challenge lite butter, which is less than ½ the fat of regular butter
1 cup cream	½ cup nonfat milk and ½ cup cooked potato or vegetables, blended for creamy thickness, or skim evaporated milk, which has a rich flavor and color, or skim powdered milk for thickness and richness

Dinners

Here are some ideas for taking typical high fat dinner meals and lowering their fat. Some of the ingredients in lasagne, beef stroganoff and hamburgers are high in fat, so we have extracted those items that can be exchanged for lower fat versions and given you the substitutions below.

For Lasagne:

INSTEAD OF THIS	TRY THIS
Whole ricotta cheese	Nonfat ricotta cheese
Whole mozzarella cheese	Lite or nonfat mozzarella cheese
One egg	¼ cup egg substitute
Sausage	½ sausage and ½ ground round or ground turkey

For Beef Stroganoff:

INSTEAD OF THIS	TRY THIS
Butter	Lite butter
Beef, sliced	Half beef, half mushrooms
Crème fraîche or sour cream	Half yogurt cheese, half sour cream or nonfat sour cream

106

For Hamburgers:

INSTEAD OF THIS	TRY THIS
Hamburger	Extra lean beef, chicken, turkey or fish
Slice of cheese	Slice of low fat cheese
Mayonnaise	Low fat mayonnaise
Avocado	Roasted bell pepper or low fat guacamole (see recipe index)

Desserts

Desserts are something we all look forward to and do not want to give up. And, the good news is we don't have to. There are lots of tasty substitutions for many of our favorite desserts. Here are some examples:

INSTEAD OF THIS	TRY THIS
Pie	Berry Crisp (see recipe index)
Ice cream	Low fat ice cream, ice milk or nonfat frozen yogurt
Chocolate Mousse	Chocolate pudding made with evaporated skim milk or a Fudgsicle
Chocolate bar	Tootsie Roll or chocolate jelly beans
Fudge sauce	Hershey's nonfat chocolate sauce or our Fudgy Cocoa Sauce (see recipe index)
Pound cake	Angel food cake

107

As an additional example of substitutions, here is a full day's low fat replacements, from breakfast to lunch to dinner, including snacks.

Savory Solutions in Making Better Choices

INSTEAD OF THIS	Grams of Fat	TRY THIS	Grams of Fat
Breakfast			
Doughnut, glazed	12	Bagel	2
Toast with butter and jelly	6	Toast with jelly	1
Granola, 1 cup	15	Bran flakes, 1 cup	1
Whole milk, 1 cup	8	Skim milk, 1 cup	0
French toast, 2 slices	12	French toast with egg substitute	2
Omelette, 3 eggs	18	Omelette, 1 yolk and 3 whites, with fresh salsa	6
Cappuccino with whole milk	4	Cappuccino with nonfat milk	0
Subtotal	**75**	**Subtotal**	**12**
Lunch			
Regular tortilla, fried in fat, filled with refried beans and cheese	24	Low fat tortilla, filled with nonfat refried beans, 1 Tbsp. green chile, ¼ oz. low fat cheese	3
Big Mac	32	Small hamburger, plain	9
Burrito, beef and bean, frozen	15	Burrito, red chile, frozen	5
Hot dog on bun with condiments	15	Hot dog, low fat on a bun with low fat condiments	6
Tuna packed in oil, 2 oz.	13	Tuna packed in water, 2 oz.	1
Milk shake, 10 oz.	10	Nonfat ice cream milk shake	0
Salad with oil and vinegar	15	Salad with nonfat dressing or lemon or rice vinegar	0
Turkey sandwich with 1 Tbsp. mayonnaise	30	Low fat turkey sandwich with mustard or nonfat mayonnaise	12
Subtotal	**154**	**Subtotal**	**36**

108

INSTEAD OF THIS		TRY THIS	
	Grams of Fat		Grams of Fat

Dinner

INSTEAD OF THIS	Grams of Fat	TRY THIS	Grams of Fat
Chicken leg, fried, 5 oz.	11	Chicken leg, baked or BBQ with skin removed and a nonfat marinade, 5 oz.	4
Fried rice, 1 cup	7	Steamed rice, 1 cup	2
Broccoli with butter	15	Broccoli with lemon	0
French fries, 10 pieces	8	Skinny French Fries, 10 pieces (see recipe index)	1
Cheese pizza, 2 slices	24	Boboli, ¼ of a 16-oz. round with tomato sauce and low fat mozzarella grated cheese	8
Shrimp, fried, 3 oz.	10	Shrimp sautéed with wine and herbs, 3 oz.	1
Subtotal	**75**	**Subtotal**	**16**

109

Snacks

INSTEAD OF THIS	Grams of Fat	TRY THIS	Grams of Fat
Peanuts, ½ cup, oil roasted	35	Orville Redenbacher's Smart Pop, 1 cup	0
Potato chips (10)	7	Low fat potato chips (10)	2
Ice cream, 1 cup	14	Frozen juice bar or nonfat ice cream	0
Chocolate candy bar	9	Jelly beans (10)	0
1 slice American cheese, 1 oz.	8	Low fat cheese, 1 oz.	4
2 chocolate chip cookies	10	1 piece angel food cake with fresh crushed strawberries and nonfat yogurt	trace
Baby Ruth, 1 bar	12	Butterscotch hard candy, 1 oz. or 5 pieces	1
Subtotal	**95**	**Subtotal**	**7**
TOTAL	**399**	**TOTAL**	**71**

Summarizing the Art of Low Fat Food Substitutions

The following is a progression of how you can substitute high fat foods with absolutely no fat to low fat products or combinations of low fat products.

1. Check out your grocery market to see what nonfat substitutes are available. For example, use Nonfat Philadelphia Cream Cheese for regular cream cheese.

2. If a nonfat substitute isn't available, use a low fat substitute. For example, for regular buttermilk, use low fat buttermilk, and for regular butter, use a light butter.

3. If neither a nonfat or low fat substitute is available, use a low fat substitute whose texture and taste is similar to the ingredient you want to replace. For example, instead of Half & Half in a baking recipe, you can combine nonfat buttermilk with vanilla yogurt to make a comparable substitute.

110

4. If you can't find anything that is a complete substitute, try a partial substitute. For example, in a dessert that calls for butter, use ½ the butter the recipe calls for and ½ of a fruit purée. This generally works quite well.

5. If your substitution deals with eggs, you can cut down on egg yolks and use more egg whites; or you can use egg substitutes which are 99% real egg products (egg whites, nonfat dry milk, lecithin). We keep one carton of egg substitute in the refrigerator at all times and if we don't use it in one week, we toss it. Egg substitutes are great for baking, stuffing and coatings. If you are making an omelette or scrambled eggs, use 1 whole egg and the rest egg whites or egg substitute. Try different egg substitutes; some are better than others. Remember, each egg yolk you eliminate is 5–6 less grams of fat, most of which is saturated.

You need to wear your Sherlock Holmes hat and bring your spy glass to the grocery store so you can be a fat detective.

As you become more familiar with low fat products, you'll see there are many substitutions at the grocery store. You need to wear your Sherlock Holmes hat and bring your spy glass to the grocery store so you can be a fat detective. You can start by cutting ½ of the fat from your own tried-and-true recipes.

The key to successful low fat cooking—at least in the beginning—is moderation, moderation, moderation. Don't try to suddenly eliminate all fat from your dishes—if you are able to eliminate ⅓ to ½ of the fat you're now consuming, you will have taken a giant step forward.

> **It is more important to gradually reduce the fat in your meals and retain good flavor and texture, than to greatly reduce or eliminate fat and end up with something tasteless and undesirable.**

111

STEP 25 — **Veggie Power**

It seems almost every day a new discovery is announced about the health-giving, healing power of vegetables. It's now widely acknowledged that they have anti-cancer properties (phytochemicals), help prevent heart attacks, prevent premature aging, and are beneficial for almost every human health problem. We know that vegetables are a great source of vitamins, minerals and fiber, plus, they have *just a trace of fat!* And we know that vegetables tend to be more nutritious than fruits.

Yet for all of this, vegetables are one of the hardest food groups for which youngsters (and sometimes spouses) can develop a taste. It is rare to find a vegetable the whole family likes . . . usually one person likes two or three choices, another will eat only peas, and another will not touch anything green.

So instead of using up a lot of space lecturing to you on how good veggies are for you, we're going to describe how to prepare vegetables that the whole family can enjoy.

> **The darker or more colorful a vegetable is, the more nutrients it has.**

We'll start by talking about color. The darker or more colorful a vegetable is, the more nutrients it has. So, where possible, you'll want to choose veggies like broccoli, spinach, carrots and tomatoes, instead of cucumbers, celery or iceberg lettuce.

Choose from the following vegetables often. They are chock-full of health-promoting phyto-chemicals and antioxidants such as Vitamin C and Beta Carotene.

GREEN	RED	YELLOW	WHITE
Broccoli	Tomatoes	Carrots	Cauliflower
Green Peppers	Red Peppers	Acorn Squash	Garlic
Spinach	Onions	Yams	
Kale, Chard		Onions	
Brussels Sprouts			
Cabbage, Bok Choy			

The more vegetables are processed, the more nutrients they lose. Fresh vegetables should be your first choice, frozen vegetables should be your second choice, and thirdly, you should choose canned vegetables.

Pre-cut, ready-to-eat veggies sold in grocery stores are an option for when you don't have time to wash and chop. Veggies packaged this way are still high in nutrients because the plastic wrapping keeps them from breathing.

> **Of the various ways of cooking vegetables, steaming and sautéing are the methods that retain the most nutrients.**

Vegetables are easy to ruin. Most people overcook them. But, cooked just right, the colors and textures are divine. In this step, we'll give you several different cooking methods to whet your appetite. These ideas will help you think of veggies as the main event instead of a side dish.

We'll start with the different methods and styles of preparing vegetables.

113

Cooking Method—Blanch

To submerge food in boiling liquid and cook to your desired doneness.

Example: Broccoli

1. Add vegetables in small amounts so the water will remain at a constant boil (if you lose the boil they will take longer to cook and lose color, texture and nutritive value).
2. Place broccoli florets in boiling water.
3. As soon as the broccoli turns bright green, remove it (anywhere from ½–3 minutes, depending on the size of the florets and the amount of water).
4. Your vegetables will keep cooking after you drain them and place them on a

serving platter, so it's best to undercook them. You can place them in cold water to stop the cooking, but we prefer to do it in one step, so we undercook them knowing they will continue to cook a little.

Cooking Method—Bake

To cook foods in an enclosed oven with circulated heat and a constant temperature. Select vegetables that take about the same amount of time to cook.

Example: Baked carrots, onions and potatoes

1. Preheat oven to 350°–375°.
2. Peel carrots and cut to a size similar to the baby onions and the baby new potatoes.
3. Skin onions, leaving the ends intact, and clean the potatoes.
4. Spray a roasting pan with olive oil.
5. Put carrots, onions and potatoes in roasting pan and spray them with oil.
6. Season with salt, pepper and garlic powder. You can also throw some rosemary in the roasting pan for a wonderful flavor, or try adding 1/2 cup of white wine. Every half hour, shake the pan and respray the ingredients so they become golden brown and don't stick.

Cook approximately 1 hour or until done.

Cooking Method—Barbeque (or BBQ)

This term is usually applied to outdoor cooking on a charcoal grill; however, barbequing can be done on indoor grills as well.

Example: Marinated vegetable barbeque

This technique gives vegetables a wonderful sweet flavor and color. Suitable vegetables:

Eggplant, sliced ½" thick the long way
New potatoes, precooked and cut in 1" slices; or if very small potatoes, keep whole

114

Carrots, the small baby ones

Baby onions

Zucchini, sliced ½" thick the long way

Sweet potatoes, precooked and cut in 1" slices

1. Immerse vegetables in this marinade mixture for 5 to 10 minutes.

   ¼ cup rice vinegar

   2 tablespoons soy sauce

   ¼ cup balsamic vinegar

   1 teaspoon garlic, minced

   1 tablespoon fresh rosemary

2. Wipe your grill with a paper towel dipped in oil so the food won't stick.

3. Spray the marinated vegetables with oil and place the sprayed side down on the BBQ.

4. Spray the other side while it's cooking, and turn vegetables when browned.

5. Cook until golden on both sides depending on size and variety.

6. Salt and pepper to taste while cooking.

Barbequed vegetables can be served hot or at room temperature.

Cooking Method—Steam

To cook by contact with steam in a covered container or perforated container placed over hot water.

Most vegetables are suitable for steaming. The water level should be low enough so that it doesn't touch the vegetables but high enough so that it doesn't boil away before the vegetables are cooked.

Example: Steamed zucchini

2 pounds zucchini, cut into small rounds

6 basil leaves

Salt and pepper to taste

115

1. Place the zucchini rounds in a steamer with the water at a boil.
2. When they turn bright green, remove them.
3. Julienne the basil leaves (cut into matchstick-size thin strips) and sprinkle them on top of the zucchini.
4. Season and serve.

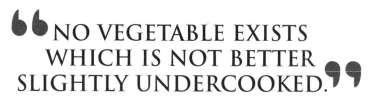

"NO VEGETABLE EXISTS WHICH IS NOT BETTER SLIGHTLY UNDERCOOKED."

–James Beard

Cooking Method—Stew

To simmer food in a small amount of liquid.

Example: Ratatouille

Ratatouille is a wonderful vegetable stew that you can eat hot or cold. You can use a variety of vegetables, but the following are traditional:

1 medium red onion, cut into ⅛'s

6 garlic cloves, finely chopped

3 Japanese eggplants, medium, sliced into ¾" thick slices (about 3 cups)

2 bell peppers cut into ¾" strips (about 2 cups)

1 pound zucchini or summer squash cut into ¾" pieces (about 2 cups)

2 pounds vine-ripened tomatoes, peeled, seeded and chopped (about 3 cups)

1 bay leaf

2 sprigs of fresh marjoram

1. Heat skillet and spray with canola or olive oil.
2. Add onion and garlic and sauté until limp.
3. Respray the pan and add eggplant and bell peppers. Sauté for 5–8 minutes until tender.
4. Next, add squash, tomatoes, bay leaf and salt and pepper to taste.

116

5. Stew over low heat for 20 minutes, until everything is tender.

6. Add the basil and marjoram just before serving. Retaste for salt and ground pepper.

Cooking Method—Sauté

To fry quickly over a moderately high heat in a pan sprayed with canola or olive oil or a minimum amount of other fat, turning or stirring frequently.

Example: Oriental Vegetable Sauté

½ yellow onion, cleaned, cut in half and then cut into thin strips

1 cup fresh mushrooms, cleaned and sliced

1 bunch broccoli, cleaned and cut into small florets

¼ cup vegetable broth

Lite soy sauce

1. Spray a large sauté pan with oil.

2. Sauté the yellow onion until it is golden.

3. Respray pan and add mushrooms. Sauté them until all the juice they release dries up.

4. Respray the pan with oil and add the broccoli florets—sauté for 2 minutes.

5. Add the vegetable broth and lite soy sauce to taste.

6. Turn the heat up for 1 minute, then serve.

117

Preparation Style—Brochette

Anything cooked on a skewer may be called a brochette.

Example: Brochette of fresh vegetables. The following are suggested veggies to use:

Small onions, no more than 1"–1½" in diameter, peeled

Red, yellow and green bell peppers, cut in 1"–1½" squares

Zucchini, 1"–1½" thick slices

Summer squash, 1"–1½" slices; if small, use whole

Mushrooms, 1" whole

Petite new potatoes, 1"–1½" slices; parboil to 3/4 done

Cherry tomatoes, whole

Basil or sage

Try to have all of the vegetables the same size so that they will cook to the same doneness.

1. Use the following marinade to brush on your brochette, or marinate for 5 to 10 minutes and use the extra marinade during cooking.

   6 tablespoons lite soy sauce

   2 tablespoons Mirin*

   2 teaspoons minced garlic

   Salt and pepper

2. Place fresh basil or fresh sage leaves on skewers (every third vegetable).

3. Wipe grill with a paper towel dipped in oil so veggies won't stick.

4. Cook on skewers until golden.

5. You can spray with oil to keep from sticking and to get a golden color.

6. Serve with brown and wild rice mixed with toasted, slivered almonds, or polenta sprinkled with Parmesan cheese.

Preparation Style—Casserole

An ovenproof cooking pot with a lid; also, the food cooked in it, which consists of more than one ingredient, usually in sauce. Considered a one-dish meal. Example: Chili Vegetable Casserole

1. Take another look at your favorite chili recipe. Leave out the beef and add ground chicken, ground turkey or textured vegetable protein. Textured vegetable protein is a meat substitute made from soybeans. It is low in fat and can be purchased at most health food stores.

2. Start by sautéing onions and garlic until golden in your sprayed sauté pan.

118

---

* *Mirin is a sweet rice wine found in most grocery stores and all Japanese grocery stores.*

3. Follow your recipe on top of the stove or put it in the oven like a vegetable chili casserole at 350°.

4. When serving, add some fresh cilantro and a dollop of nonfat sour cream to individual servings.

Preparation Style—Parchment

A tough, usually translucent, paper for lining baking pans or wrapping food to be prepared in papillote (cooked in a bag or packet).

Example: Shiitake Mushroom Potato in Papillote (single serving)

3 shiitake mushrooms, or 3 regular mushrooms

3 or 4 small red potatoes, cut in 1/4's or 1/6's

1 sheet parchment paper 11" by 16"

3 or 4 unpeeled garlic cloves, smashed

1 fresh marjoram sprig

1 fresh sage leaf

Olive spray

Dry white wine

1. Preheat oven to 400°.

2. Remove mushroom stems, and cut into 1" pieces.

3. Lay the parchment on a work surface and place mushroom, potatoes and fresh herbs in center.

4. Spray oil over vegetables; add a splash of wine, salt and pepper.

5. Fold parchment over vegetables so the edges of the paper meet.

6. Roll the parchment tightly along the edges, forming a semicircle as you go.

7. When you reach the end, tuck the last corner snugly under itself to seal the packet.

8. Place on a baking sheet and bake for 20 minutes or more, until done.

Variations: leeks, scallions or a combination of vegetables with similar cooking times.

119

Preparation Style—Stuffed

A vegetable (for example, bell pepper, tomato, squash or eggplant), cooked or uncooked, from which you remove the soft meaty material in the center, prepare a filling, stuff the vegetable and cook it. Some vegetables, such as tomatoes, can be stuffed and served without cooking.

Example: Stuffed Yellow and Red Bell Peppers

6 bell peppers, 3 yellow and 3 red

1 cup fresh corn, cooked, stripped from the cob (about 2 small ears)

1 cup cooked baby shrimp or 1 cup of any of the following: lean ground chicken or turkey (cooked), textured vegetable protein

1 cup fine bread crumbs

1 whole egg and 3 egg whites, or 8 ounces of egg substitute

2 ribs celery, cut in ¼'s

1 yellow onion medium, cut in ¼'s

2 cloves of garlic

¼ cup parsley leaves, washed

½ cup mushrooms

2 green scallions, cut in ¼'s

½ cup skim evaporated milk

Salt, pepper and garlic salt

1. Cut the top off the bell peppers and clean out any white veins and seeds.

2. Place the bell peppers in boiling water for 3 minutes.

3. Then place the bell peppers in a sprayed baking pan.

4. Place corn, shrimp (or meat, etc.), bread crumbs and eggs in a bowl.

5. Put celery, onion, garlic, parsley, mushrooms and scallions in a food processor and pulse 20 times until chopped, medium-fine.

6. Sauté this mixture in a sprayed sauté pan until golden.

7. Add the evaporated milk to the pan and keep the heat high. Then scrape the pan to retain the pan brownings.

8. Add this mixture to the corn, shrimp (or meat or textured vegetable protein), bread and egg, adding the seasonings and stirring to blend.

9. Stuff the peppers with this mixture and cook in a preheated oven at 375° for 1 hour.

10. Ten minutes before they are finished cooking, put a tablespoon of your favorite red sauce on top of each bell pepper (optional); finish cooking.

11. When serving, cut peppers in half and serve ½ a red one and ½ a yellow one, filling side down on the plate.

This recipe works well as a fish, meat or meatless dish.

Preparation Style—Phyllo

Leaf-thin sheets of dough made from flour and water. Use layered with sweet or savory fillings. Also spelled filo. (In either case, it's pronounced fee-low.)

Example: Phyllo with Spinach and Mushrooms

2 bags spinach, washed and stemmed

1 cup mushrooms, cleaned and finely chopped

½ cup white wine

1 teaspoon garlic, chopped

2 teaspoons fresh marjoram chopped, or 1 teaspoon dried

¼ teaspoon fresh nutmeg, ground or 1/8 teaspoon dried

⅓ cup raisins

1 tablespoon yellow onion, chopped

¼ cup water

½ pound fat-free phyllo dough

8 tablespoons fine bread crumbs, no seasoning

121

1 tablespoon parsley, chopped

1 egg white, beaten

1. Add the wine to a sauté pan and simmer spinach until wilted.
2. Drain completely by putting in a strainer and press out excess liquid with a cereal bowl.
3. Spray a sauté pan and sauté the garlic and mushrooms.
4. Add the spinach, garlic salt, pepper and chopped marjoram to the garlic mushroom sauté.
5. In a blender, place nutmeg, raisins, onion and water. Blend to purée.
6. Preheat oven to 350°.

122

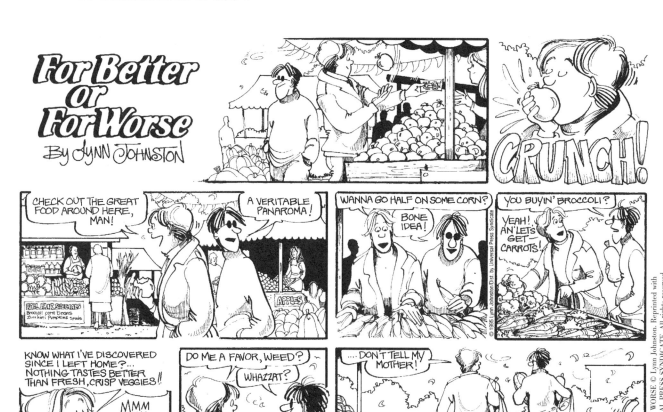

7. Lay out one sheet of phyllo, being careful to cover with a damp cloth while working.
8. Brush phyllo lightly with the raisin/onion mixture, covering entire piece of phyllo in a thin layer.
9. Next, sprinkle approximately 2 teaspoons of the bread crumbs over the raisin mixture.
10. Spread a thin layer of the spinach/garlic/mushroom mixture.
11. Sprinkle ¼ of the parsley over spinach layer.
12. Repeat with the next 4 sheets of phyllo.
13. On sheet 5 don't cover with raisin/onion mixture, bread crumbs, or spinach mixture. Instead, spray sheet with a light mist of olive oil, leaving a 1" border.
14. Roll the phyllo tightly lengthwise like a jelly roll; use the raisin mixture to seal seam ends.
15. Fold ends down under to prevent filling from leaking.
16. Spray a cookie sheet with canola or olive oil and brush the jelly roll with egg white and spray with oil.
17. Bake for 30 minutes. Allow 10 minutes to cool. Cut in 1" thick diagonal slices to serve.

123

Preparation Style—Enchilada

A Mexican-American dish of a tortilla stuffed with a mixture of vegetables and/or meat, cheese, onions and covered with an enchilada sauce.

Example: Chicken Vegetable Enchilada

4 chicken breasts, without skins or bone (optional)
1–2 cups of cooked vegetables
10 flour or corn tortillas
4-ounce can of green chiles
6 ounces of low fat cheese

1 can enchilada sauce
1 can chopped tomatoes in juice
½ can chopped olives
1 9" x 12" Pyrex dish

1. Heat your oven to 350°.

2. Season the chicken breasts and bake at 350° for 30 minutes.

3. Cook the tortillas on each side in a medium-hot sauté pan (no oil spray necessary).

4. Shred the chicken and divide it into 10 piles.

5. Put a portion of chicken, chopped chiles, vegetables and cheese onto a tortilla, roll it up, fold the ends under and place it in the Pyrex dish. Do the same for each tortilla, leaving some of the cheese aside.

6. When all the tortillas are filled, mix the cans of enchilada sauce and chopped tomatoes and then pour this sauce over the tops of the filled tortillas.

7. Sprinkle the chopped olives over the sauce, and then sprinkle the cheese over the olives.

8. Bake in the oven at 350° for 40–45 minutes.

9. Serve with a dollop of nonfat sour cream and fresh salsa on top.

124

We've given you twelve different ways to prepare vegetables—from simple steaming and sautéing to the more sophisticated brochette or stuffed methods. There are many more ways, limited only by your imagination.

We feel strongly about including lots of vegetables in your diet. We believe great benefits come from eating vegetables. We call it Veggie Power. The Food Pyramid tells us to have 3–6 servings of vegetables each day, and studies of health and longevity around the world show that, time after time, people who eat a variety of vegetables each day live longer and healthier lives—and veggies have just a trace of fat!

When vegetables become a large portion of your daily food intake, the amount of fat you are eating invariably decreases, with the inevitable result of weight loss if you are overweight.

A Brief Word from Joan

As a child, I was never told there was a bad vegetable and my mom cooked everything from parsnips to peas. I think it's important that parents don't taint their children's attitudes by passing on their own vegetable prejudices. My own grandchildren grab vegetables as they would any other treats, at least in part because no one has told them they wouldn't like them. In fact, it's the broccoli (we call broccoli florets "trees") that's eaten off the plate first, before the meat! "Wow," I say to them, "you ate all your trees! You're going to grow big and tall!"

Wow, you ate all your trees! You're going to grow big and tall!

125

Vegetables abound in the kitchens of my extended family members. Having vegetables around as snacks helps. The children grab some when they see them on the table.

I hope you'll experiment with our vegetable recipes and your own. And I hope you'll pass on this positive attitude toward veggies to your children, your spouse and your friends.

The story of herbs and spices reaches back to the earliest records of human activity where they were used not only as flavorings, but as medicines, good luck charms, fragrant air fresheners, decorative bouquets and romantic lures. Until recent times, they were grown in every household garden, and their many uses were common knowledge to homemakers. But as we have gone to canned foods, frozen dinners, more meat and fast-food restaurants in the last 30–40 years, we have lost this wonderful gift of good eating. But now we must pay more attention to cooking with less meat and less fat, so we're looking for new ways to enhance the flavor of foods. Herbs and spices, the magical seasonings, are one of the keys to this cooking renaissance.

Fresh vs. Dried

126

For us, there is no debate about this—we love fresh herbs and, whenever possible, we choose them over dried ones. Not only are the flavor and aroma of fresh herbs finer for cooking, but keeping a vase of fresh herbs on the counter allows their wonderful scent to spread through the kitchen. Sometimes we mix them in a bouquet with fresh flowers; often, they are pretty enough by themselves. Also, when we are entertaining, a nice treat for our guests is to place a small vase of herbs on each table. Many of the common herbs—basil, mint, sage, rosemary, fennel and thyme—are available fresh year-round, so there is no need to buy them dried.

Spices, on the other hand, grow mostly in tropical areas and are only available locally in dried form. But most spice distributors do a good job of quick-drying and then packaging them in airtight containers that seal in the flavor.

Tasting and Smelling

Get to know the herbs and spices you'll be using. If you don't have an herb garden, buy a sprig of each fresh herb offered at your market. When you're back home and the groceries are put away, test them one at a time. Rub a leaf between your fingers to release all the taste and aroma, or cut off a thin slice of root. Place it on your tongue and press your tongue up against the roof of your mouth (more taste receptors are engaged when food is pressed against them). Breathe in to catch the aroma. Then swallow.

> ❝ **LAUGHTER IS THE BEST SEASONING THERE IS.** ❞
>
> —*Barbara Kafka*

Be aware of the several taste sensations you are picking up. Think about the taste . . . make some mental comparisons of this taste to others you know, and file this new knowledge away in your memory. Do this with each of the fresh herbs you've bought. When time permits, also try this with the dried herbs and spices in your pantry. Gradually, you'll build up a mental library of each herb and spice, and this will help you decide which ones to use in preparing dishes.

127

From Your Garden

What a delight it is to have your own herb garden! Whenever you need herbs, you simply step outside and pick them. They are also attractive along garden walkways and they make good border plants.

Most herbs are easy to grow. Just choose a sheltered spot with lots of sun, preferably on a slope or other spot with good drainage. If they don't receive several hours of direct sunlight during the day, their flavor and aroma will be weak.

If possible, choose a spot near your kitchen door—when the weather is bad you can just pop out and back in again. Even in climates with extreme temperatures, some herbs will remain green year-round. However, you'll want to make sure you have a steady supply, by either drying some or freezing them.

If you have an herb garden, choose a sunny day for collecting, and pick leaves around midmorning, when the leaves are free of dew. An herb plant is perfect for harvesting when the flower buds are just beginning to open.

If you want to use them while they are fresh, place intact stems and leaves in a vase of water. For air-drying, you can tie a bunch of stems together and hang them upside-down. For large-leafed herbs, remove the leaves from the stems and place the leaves on a drying screen so that there is air circulation all around them. To retain the most flavor and aroma, dry your herbs inside in a warm, shady place that has good air circulation. Depending on the temperature and humidity inside, it may take up to two weeks for them to dry completely. The herbs are dry when the leaves crumble easily in your hand.

For quick drying, you can use your oven or microwave. To dry herbs in your oven, place them on the oven shelf on a brown paper bag, and set the oven to the lowest temperature (which should be around 100°). Every 10–15 minutes, turn the leaves over. Leave the oven door slightly ajar. Drying takes about 1 hour.

To microwave herbs, place a layer of leaves between two paper towels. Heat them on the high setting for one minute and then check them. Continue for 30-second intervals until they are completely dry. CAUTION: If your microwave oven does not have a rotating tray, check the leaves more frequently, since hot spots can burn the leaves quickly.

From the Store

Even if you have an herb garden, you'll want to stock your pantry with a more complete selection of dried herbs and spices than you can grow. First check to see what fresh herbs and spices your local supermarket, farmer's market or health food store offers. The rest you'll have to buy in dried form. For your initial collection, we recommend anise seed, basil, bay leaf, caraway seed, chili powder, cinnamon, coriander, dill, ginger, marjoram and nutmeg. Buying herbs and spices in small tins or bottles can be expensive. If you have some small containers at home that have an airtight seal, try going to your local health food or bulk food store and buying *small* amounts in bulk.

Storage

To retain all the wonderful flavor and aroma of herbs, here's what to do: For herbs you have dried (or bought in bulk from the store), make sure they are completely dry. Then remove the leaves from the stems and place the dried leaves in airtight containers. Store them in a cool, dry, dark place. They'll retain their flavor and aroma for about six months.

To freeze most herbs you first have to blanch them (exceptions are basil, chives and dill). For small sprigs, leave them intact. For larger leaves, take the leaves off the stems. Place the sprigs or leaves in a colander and pour boiling water over them for a few seconds. Make sure the hot water contacts all the leaves. Then spread them out to dry on a towel. When they are dry, transfer them to a dish and place them in your freezer. Freeze them for 2–3 hours. Then transfer them once more into freezer-safe containers and place them in the freezer. Don't use soft plastic bags as the herbs are likely to be bruised or crushed. When you're ready to use them, remove whatever amount you need, but not more than you need—you can't refreeze them once they have been thawed.

For storing fresh garlic, place it in a ceramic container and keep it in a cool, dry place. Don't store garlic in the refrigerator—it may sprout and turn bitter.

Fresh ginger is best kept frozen without drying. Wrap it tightly in plastic and, when you need some, grate it right from the frozen root without thawing it.

If you are drying and bottling your own herbs, remember to add the date underneath the name of the herb. When stored properly, dried herbs will retain their flavor and aroma for about one year.

Using Herbs and Spices

Always use fresh herbs if you possibly can—you'll love the superb flavor and aroma they add to your dish. When you are first learning to use herbs and spices, use about ¾ of what the recipe calls for, and taste it. You can always

129

> **Remember, herbs are meant to enhance the flavor of food, not to mask it.**

add more, but you can't remove it once it's in. Remember, herbs are meant to enhance the flavor of food, not to mask it.

Herbs and spices are much more compact when dried than when fresh, so if a recipe calls for 1 teaspoon of dried herb, that's the equivalent of 3 teaspoons of fresh (finely chopped).

With herbs, a general rule is to use 1 teaspoon of dried herbs for every 2–4 servings. That's just to give you some idea of the amount you'll probably need. Again, taste, taste, taste! There's no substitute for your skilled palate.

Here are a few tips to remember:

- Always use fresh herbs, if available.
- Use 3 times as much fresh herb as dry.
- Start out with less than the recipe calls for—then taste and add as desired.
- Allow herbs to soak in the recipe liquid for 5–10 minutes before adding the other ingredients. This allows the flavors to develop.
- When a recipe calls for adding herbs to hot liquids, rub them in your hands to release the aromatic oils—then add them.
- Hot liquids evaporate some of the aromatic oils in herbs. To get the best of both flavor and aroma, divide the herbs in half. Put half of them into the soup or stew at the beginning and keep the other half out until about the last 10 minutes—then add them.
- For salads, you can add fresh or dried herbs to the salad dressing (allow it to sit for a while before serving). With fresh herbs, try chopping them into small pieces and tossing them directly into the salad.

130

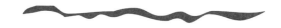

If you're creating on your own (which we hope you'll do), here's a chart that suggests which herbs go well with various foods.

HERB AND FOOD COMBINATIONS

Herb	Beef	Chicken	Fish	Lamb	Pork	Egg	Salad	Vegetable	Pasta Sauce	Sauce	Soup	Dessert	Tea
Anise												X	X
Basil*		X	X				X	X	X	X	X		
Bay/Laurel	X		X		X						X	X	
Caraway					X		X				X		
Chives*		X	X			X	X	X	X		X		
Cilantro*		X	X		X		X	X		X	X		
Coriander	X	X	X	X	X						X		
Dill*		X	X				X	X		X	X		
Fennel		X	X	X			X	X			X		
Horseradish	X									X			
Lemongrass*	X	X	X			X				X			
Marjoram*	X	X	X		X	X	X	X					
Mint*			X		X		X	X		X	X	X	X
Nasturtium							X				X		
Oregano	X	X	X			X		X			X		
Parsley*		X	X	X	X	X	X	X	X	X	X		
Rosemary*	X	X	X	X	X		X			X			
Sage*	X	X	X		X				X	X	X		
Savory		X			X	X	X				X		
Tarragon*		X	X	X			X	X		X			
Thyme*		X	X	X	X	X			X	X	X		

* Can be found fresh at most grocery stores.

Herbal Vinegars

To make your own herbal vinegar, start with 2 cups of white, red or rice vinegar and start adding small amounts of your favorite herbs. Remember, taste, taste, taste!

Here are some suggestions:

1. Basil, oregano, 1 clove garlic (minced or left whole)
2. Lemon slices, thyme or dill
3. Rosemary, marjoram, orange slices
4. Garlic, parsley, sage, thyme

Flavor Boosters

And finally, here's a list of flavor boosters that should be in every kitchen:

- Black pepper
- Butter
- Cayenne pepper
- Crushed red pepper flakes
- Garlic
- Lemon
- Lime
- Mustard, natural ground
- Olive oil
- Onion
- Orange zest
- Red pepper
- Salsa
- Salt
- Scallions
- Shallots
- Soy sauce
- Spices (Allspice, Cinnamon, Clove, Cumin, Ginger, Nutmeg, etc.)
- Sun-dried tomatoes
- Vinegar
- White pepper
- Wine for cooking

As you become used to cooking with herbs and spices, a whole new world of culinary delight will unfold for you. The combinations of tasty flavors and heady aromas are almost endless. Experiment over and over, and you'll begin to accumulate your own storehouse of great recipes.

And then you can share them with your friends.

132

PART SIX

Your Food Lifestyle

STEP 27 — **Replacing Bad Food Habits
with Good Ones**

"WE ARE WHAT WE REPEATEDLY DO."
—*Aristotle*

All of us have feelings about food and eating that we have learned over the years. Food is a symbol of many things for different people—love, celebration, reward, a bond with family or a boredom reliever. In order for us to change poor eating habits, we need to examine our lifelong relationship with food.

Food habits play a big role in what we eat and when we eat. Habits are funny things: in theory, we can change them instantly by merely willing ourselves to do so, but in practice they are stubborn—they cling to us with a lot of tenacity and resist being changed. Let's begin by taking a look at some common food habits:

Part 1: Addictions

1. Do you ever open your refrigerator just to see if something desirable is inside?

2. After completing some task do you reward yourself with food?

3. Do you eat to feel better when you're bored, unhappy or tense?

In order for us to change poor eating habits, we need to examine our life-long relationship with food.

133

4. Do you eat more than you normally would because you are reading or watching TV?

5. Do you "even out" your last bits of food on your plate (e.g., some of your drink is left so you get a bit more solid food to go with it, and vice versa)?

6. Do you feel that you have to finish everything on your plate, even if you're no longer hungry?

7. Do you eat because it is mealtime, even if you're not hungry?

8. Do you munch on things when you're preparing food?

9. Do you eat pretty well during the week, but indulge on holidays and weekends?

10. Do you find that you need to constantly sip a drink or snack while you're working?

11. Do you rationalize that it is okay to "pig out" if you're eating at someone else's house or at a party?

Part 2: Temptations

12. Do you greatly enjoy cooking for others?

13. Do you frequently attend events and activities that center around food?

14. Do people you associate with offer you overly rich foods (often saying, "One bite won't hurt")?

15. Do friends and/or family members try to please you by bringing you fatty treats?

The higher the number of "yes" answers to the above questions, the greater the danger of your being or becoming a food addict. In truth, most of us are food addicts. And the most effective way to stop being a food addict is to become more aware of what you're doing.

Eating Triggers

Have you ever noticed yourself staring blindly into your refrigerator? Do you sometimes look at the clock and think you need to eat lunch just because it's the noon hour? Have you ever gone to the movies and ordered popcorn with butter, even though you just ate dinner? These are examples of *eating triggers*. They are events or stimuli that so often lead to poor eating habits.

Eating triggers can be external or internal. External triggers involve your senses of smell, sight and sound, and are usually easy to identify. Internal triggers are more complex. They center around moods and feelings, such as anger, boredom, anxiety and self-gratification.

We need to become more aware of what triggers us to eat poorly, so that we can replace these undesirable habits with new, healthy ones.

Awareness

Awareness is the first step to changing behavior. You can't change behavior that you're either unaware of or that you're denying. One good way to enhance your awareness of how you are eating is to keep a journal or food diary and to have visible reminders to help keep you on track, such as notes to drink glasses of water and logs to count fat grams. Once you are aware of the triggers and habits that interfere with your good intentions, you need to interrupt or stop them and move on to the next step of behavior change, which is substitution.

135

Substitution

Substitution is the act of choosing and executing some desirable alternative behavior in place of an undesirable one, such as choosing nonfat frozen yogurt in place of ice cream or taking a pleasant walk instead of having dessert. You can make substitution work better if you determine, ahead of time, several substitute actions. One way to do this is to have

Awareness is the first step to changing behavior.

a list of alternatives prepared for the times when you are tempted, so that right at the moment of temptation you have some satisfying options available. Prepare this list *now!*

Practice, Practice, Practice

The final step to behavior change is lots of practice. Don't expect to change poor eating habits overnight. It took you many years to develop them, and it will take practice and patience to change them. Research has shown that it takes 15 days to a month (consecutively) to begin to see a change in behavior. Some poor habits may take up to several months to change.

> 66 NOT TO GO BACK
> IS SOMEWHAT TO
> ADVANCE AND MEN
> MUST WALK, AT LEAST,
> BEFORE THEY DANCE. 99
>
> *—Alexander Pope*

136

Learning Positive Habits

As you become more proficient at replacing bad habits with good ones, the previous list of addictive food habits can now be changed to look like this more idealized one:

1. You no longer feel compelled to eat the last piece of food on your plate.

2. You pay attention to what your body is signaling you, and you eat if you are hungry—not just because it is time to eat.

3. You have stopped opening the refrigerator out of boredom.

4. You have learned to give yourself satisfying non-food rewards.

5. When you feel stressed, angry, depressed or bored, you look into your feeling and no longer automatically eat in order to feel better.

6. You have learned to taste when necessary—but not snack—while you're cooking.

7. You can now enjoy sporting events and movies without having to snack during them.

8. Instead of starving yourself so you can "pig out" at a party later in the day, now you have learned to eat moderately ahead of time.

9. You have stopped watching TV or reading while you eat, or, if you still do, you limit yourself to a certain amount of time for eating—and then you stop when your time is up.

10. You now understand that weekends, holidays and other special occasions are not an excuse for bingeing or eating foods that you are avoiding.

11. You have learned how to celebrate the completion of a project by pampering yourself; buying yourself a gift, going out with a friend, etc., and you no longer feel the need to overeat in order to celebrate.

Developing good food habits is rewarding in many ways. As you are more and more able to replace bad habits with good ones, you'll not only reap the benefits of permanent weight loss, good health and increased energy—you'll have a sense of accomplishment and you'll have the wonderful satisfaction of being in charge of yourself.

137

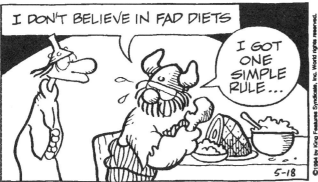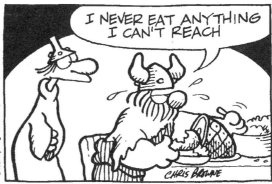

Reprinted with special permission of King Features Syndicate.

It's good to be a snacker. Most research suggests eating smaller meals more often is healthier than eating three or fewer large meals a day. It makes sense to keep feeding your engine all day long instead of overloading it at meal times and letting it starve at other times. Also, you burn calories more efficiently when you have several smaller meals. When you miss a meal your body interprets this to mean there may be a food shortage coming, so it begins to conserve fat to protect you from starving. (Remember what happens with fasting in Step 5.) By eating large meals with many hours separating them, you will retain more weight for the same amount of calories eaten. So the objective is to eat frequently and moderately.

> **The objective is to eat frequently and moderately.**

Our model is to have three meals a day with two or more snack times. If you tend to have early dinners, like at 5:30 or 6:00 P.M., then you may want a snack around 8:00 or 9:00 P.M. If, on the other hand, your dinner meal is normally 7:30 to 8:00 P.M., you will want your snack around 4:00 or 5:00 P.M. Or, if your have a different schedule, plan your own snack times—but plan them! It's okay to spontaneously grab a handful of something healthy at odd moments, but planning your snack times helps you to snack smart and to avoid overeating at meal times.

PLAN A (Late Dinner)	PLAN B (Early Dinner)	PLAN C (Your Own Plan)
Breakfast	Breakfast	_____
Snack	**Snack**	_____
Lunch	Lunch	_____
Snack	Dinner	_____
Dinner	**Snack**	_____

138

What about the quality of your snacks? If you're in a rush (who isn't?) and you miss lunch or you're starved and can't wait until you get home, you're tempted to go for whatever is nearby and quick. For example:

- Stopping at the bakery for a maple bar
- Stopping by the grocery store for a candy bar and diet coke (Nice paradox, isn't it—candy bar and *diet* coke?)
- Buying candy or high fat chips from a vending machine
- Stopping at a fast food place for some French fries

These are moments of stress. You're feeling hungry and you want something—now! So here's something very important to remember.

> **If you have good choices available at times of stress, you will select the good choices. If good choices are not available at times of stress, you will make bad choices.**

139

So let's look at some ways in which we can have good snacks available at moments of hunger stress.

Snack Storage

Why is it a good idea to put healthy snacks in one place? Because you will have preselected a variety of healthy, satisfying, low fat snacks from which you can choose. It's when you begin searching for something satisfying from all the other foods at home that you get into trouble. So keep all your snacks in one cupboard. Keep a constant supply of 5–10 low fat snacks you enjoy. There is so much on the market now that you can always buy new treats to test. You will find

Keep your snacks in one cupboard.

there are a few tried-and-true snacks you will buy over and over again. This cupboard is for the whole family, so buy new things for them to try as well. Select a variety of snacks everyone likes regardless of their age.

Keep the nonfat snacks on the lowest shelf because it's easiest to reach and put the less healthy treats nearer to the top. If you reach for the first shelf 80 percent of the time, then you are making the best choices 80 percent of the time. Even if you choose a snack from a higher shelf, it will still be better than a candy bar.

Fresh fruit snacks shouldn't be kept hidden away. They should always be available in a big bowl on the kitchen table or in a refrigerator drawer.

Try to keep a large bowl of mixed, low fat cereal someplace in the family room or kitchen for anyone to grab a handful when a snack attack hits. (There is a delicious low fat recipe for this in the recipe section.)

Have a drawer in your refrigerator filled with carrots, celery or other snackable veggies that have been cleaned and cut into convenient pieces. Keep a nonfat dip in the same drawer.

Another good place for snacks is the freezer. Keep a supply of fruit juice bars, 1-fat-gram fudge bars, frozen nonfat yogurt and yogurt bars on hand for something cold and sweet that is healthy. The same rules apply when you're away from home.

Keep at least two snacks in your car and, if you work outside the home, keep several at your office.

Remember, you want to eat mostly from the bottom of the Food Pyramid, so stick to complex carbohydrates for your snacks (pretzels, bagels, low fat crackers, cereal, vegetables, fruit, etc.), since they are absorbed slowly into the bloodstream, giving you both sustained energy and a feeling of being full. On a higher shelf in your snack cupboard, there may be some nonfat sugars, such as licorice. Although the nonfat part is good (remember that simple sugar provides no nutritive value, only calories), the sugar in the licorice is absorbed quickly, which causes your blood sugar to rise, your pancreas to pump out more insulin to return your blood sugar to normal, and then your blood sugar to fall to an even lower level than before you started. That's why you crave more of it when you eat high-sugar foods. So the licorice tasted good, but you still feel hungry and your body is working on lowering your blood sugar *instead of burning fat.*

Liquid snacks can also be very satisfying. In the summer it's nice to enjoy a low fat, fruit milk shake for a snack (see Drinks in recipes section). It's probably worth repeating here that you should drink plenty of water all during the day. Some people have no problem drinking eight 8-ounce glasses of water each day; for others it's a chore. Nowadays, there are lots of no-sugar, flavored bottled waters to choose from. One way to insure that you get plenty of water is to put ½ cup of cranberry juice into ½ gallon of water, and refrigerate it for use during the day. Try whatever works for you and helps you to meet your water quota. We recommend that you drink eight 8-ounce glasses of water each day.

Now, here's a short list of tasty, healthy snacks to help you plan for your snack attacks.

141

A Short List of Great Snacks

- ½ toasted bagel with nonfat flavored yogurt, topped with fruit
- ½ toasted bagel with fruit jelly or jam and a glass of nonfat milk
- Air-popped popcorn, sprinkled or sprayed with a nonfat seasoning

- Salads with kidney and garbanzo beans, leftover veggies, shrimp, scallions and nonfat dressings
- Miso soup (see Soups in recipes section)
- Chicken broth with noodles, egg whites, petite peas, and sliced mushrooms
- Hot chocolate, a nonfat brand
- Pretzels, all shapes and sizes, low fat and nonfat
- Tortilla chips, nonfat or low fat, with salsa or bean dip
- Flour tortillas, low fat, warmed, with nonfat refried beans, green chiles, green onions, low fat cheese
- Whole wheat bagel with nonfat cream cheese and lox
- Baked potato, with nonfat sour cream and green onions
- Corn tortillas, low fat, warmed, with salsa or bean dip
- Corn on the cob (with nonfat seasoning if desired)
- Baked yam or sweet potato (cook several ahead and keep as a sweet snack in refrigerator)
- Canned corn heated with a dollop of nonfat sour cream and fresh salsa
- Vegetable soup
- A plain pizza crust, with fresh tomatoes and low fat cheese added

When a sweet-tooth snack attack occurs and fruit just won't do, have a few helpings of licorice, jelly beans, hard candy or other nonfat confections—but keep them on the highest shelf in your snack cupboard!

Here's a summary of the things you should do for smart snacking:

- Preplan your snacks if possible, and establish between-meal snack times to suit your schedule.
- Designate a snack cupboard. Let the whole family decide what should be in it.

142

- Keep a bowl of fresh fruit and a bowl of low fat cereal in the kitchen or family room.
- Keep a drawer of snack-size, cut veggies and a nonfat dip in your refrigerator.
- Keep a pitcher or small bottles of drinking water in your refrigerator or pantry at all times.
- Have several low fat snacks at your office.
- Keep a couple of healthy snacks in your car.

And be sure to read the Appetizers & Snacks section in the recipes.

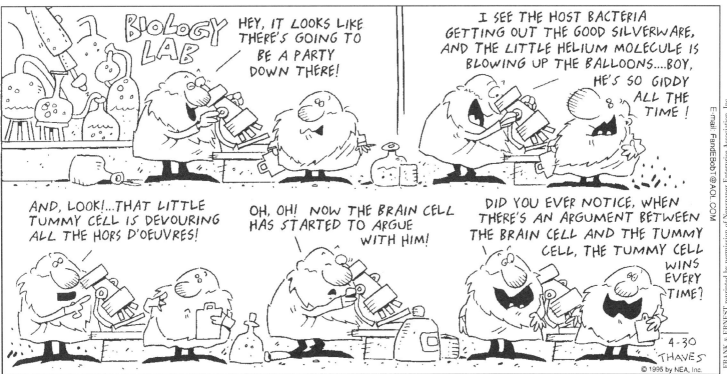

STEP 29 — **Dining, Traveling and Entertaining**

Life is full of situations with family and friends that are associated with eating. When you plan ahead and make wise choices, you don't have to miss out on the good times. Here are some strategies which will help you adjust your eating to any situation.

Dining Out

You and your friends open the menu, and you are suddenly faced with a tempting variety of . . . what? Fettucini Alfredo, lobster in Newburg sauce, baked potato with butter and sour cream—some of the most fat-filled dishes imaginable. What is it with these restaurants? Are they deliberately trying to sabotage your weight-loss program? It can certainly seem like it.

Your skinny friend who eats enough for two and who's never weighed over 95 pounds in her whole life orders a salad that will be smothered with rich Thousand Island dressing, plus a stack of toast soaked in garlic butter. Her husband goes for the prime rib plate with a double order of French fries.

And now the pressure's on you. You survey the entire menu, trying to find something that will be low fat and satisfying at the same time. Where is it? Where is it? It would be so easy just to give up and order the club sandwich with bacon.

The others are politely waiting for you, smiling patiently. The tension mounts. Then the waitress says, "Need a few more minutes, sweetie? I'll be right back."

You are saved by the bell, but the struggle goes on.

> **66 THE TROUBLE WITH EATING ITALIAN FOOD IS THAT FIVE OR SIX DAYS LATER YOU'RE HUNGRY AGAIN. 99**
>
> *–George Miller*

How many times have we all been in this situation? And it happens over and over again. Is it possible to prepare for this threat? What strategy can you employ? Is there anything at all you can do?

144

Well, yes, there are some things. They don't ensure victory, but they certainly help. For example:

> **Always ask for sauces, butter and dressings in a separate dish on the side.**

- Have a bowl of cereal or a veggie or fruit snack before leaving home to take the edge off your appetite.
- Have you been to the restaurant before? If so, you probably remember what they have. Even if it's a new restaurant, decide beforehand what types of dishes you will consider ordering. Do as much decision-making as you possibly can before you get to the restaurant, and have a few acceptable items in mind when you arrive.
- Don't be afraid to be assertive. If you're unsure, ask how items are prepared. Ask the waitress if she can recommend any low fat substitutes. Most restaurants will want to please you, so don't be afraid to ask for special treatment. For example, ask for baked potato without the butter, or hot cocoa without the whipped cream, and *always* ask for sauces, butter and dressings in a separate dish on the side.
- Order first so you won't be tempted by the choices of your companions.
- Try ordering a couple of appetizers (low fat, of course), instead of an entree . . . perhaps a shrimp or crab salad, small pizza, antipasto plate (hold the salami). Or, a low fat soup with salad and nonbuttered rolls makes a nice combination.
- Stop when you've had enough, regardless of how much is left on the plate. To ease your loss, ask for a doggie bag for your leftovers and think of how much you'll enjoy eating it at home, when you're hungry.
- At a party buffet, if they offer a choice of plate size, use the smaller one. Take small portions of many low fat dishes. Sorry, no refills.
- At a nice restaurant, eat the bread while waiting for your dinner selection—bread is one of your best choices. Limit yourself to one piece and leave the butter off.

145

• If you drink alcohol, limit yourself to one drink. A dry white- or red-wine spritzer is your best bet because it is low in calories.

Doing Fast Foods Right

You're 10 minutes into the 45-minute drive home—and you're starving. The road you're on is lined with fast food spots . . . you probably pass twenty-five or thirty of them on the way home. And it's so tempting: fries, shakes, tacos, burgers, onion rings, fried chicken! All you have to do is pull off the road and up to a drive-through window.

Then you remember that you have a snack box in the car, on the floor on the passenger side. You check it out—empty! Darn it, you forgot to refill it at the beginning of the week.

So there you are, and you're passing fast food places right and left. You really want something to nibble on or to sip . . . something to keep you company on the way home. So what do you do?

Here's something to try. Make up a list of all the fast food spots along your commute drive, in your neighborhood, etc. If you have been to each of them before and you know all the items they serve; fine. If not, stop in and check them out. Each of them will probably have a few items that are low fat. For example, salads with low fat dressing, "lite" tacos, plain baked potatoes, broiled chicken sandwiches, iced tea, diet soda, etc.

Then make a list of the items you can, in good conscience, get at each place. Make extra copies of your list in case you lose one. Keep a copy in your car at all times. You also might want to keep one, folded up, in your purse for when you are driving with someone else.

Promise yourself that if you do stop at a fast food place, you'll order only those items on your low fat list. Why don't you make up your list now?

Now when you have a terrible craving on the way home, check your list and

146

look at your options. You'll find that having some options, by itself, will relieve some of the pressure you feel to eat. Then, if you still want to stop, choose the fast food place of your choice, pull off the road, and get ready to order with the firm conviction that you are going to do two things: get your snack and keep your promise!

On the Job

It's only 10:15 A.M., but it feels like you've already put in ten hours—and you're hungry. Some of the other employees have snacks stored in the company kitchen, but by the time you get the kids off to school and help your husband get out the door on time, it's all you can do to get yourself to work.

You gave up smoking two years ago, and after that agony, it's unthinkable to light up again—so that's out. What's left? The vending machines! Packets of Famous Amos cookies, nacho chips, M&M's and a token "health bar" that tastes like recycled oatmeal.

You search in your purse for coins or single dollar bills. There aren't any quarters but you have one single bill. Without thinking further, you rush to the machine, breathless, and you choose—M&M's—but . . . the machine won't accept your bill. You straighten the edges and try again. But no matter what you do . . . no M&M's. No nothing.

Once again, you have been saved by the bell, and you slink back to your desk, suffering unimaginably. Then, in the bottom of a desk drawer you find a single piece of two-year-old Spearmint gum—and you grab it!

Most of us have been in this situation, and, once again, we need a strategy. Here are a few tips for hunger attacks at the office:

- Each night, before a work day, check your purse and make sure you don't have change for the vending machines. (In fact, try not to go near them at all.)
- Choose one day each week for stocking your desk with low fat snacks.

147

- Prepare your own low fat lunch the night before a work day.
- Use part of your work break for a brisk walk.
- Keep a container of water, tea or other low calorie drink at your desk and drink from it throughout the day.

Traveling

- Investigate your airline's special meals when you buy your tickets. Salad plates, seafood platters and vegetarian entrees are now available to choose from, but be careful: "vegetarian" doesn't necessarily mean low fat. They can have lots of cheese and butter.
- If you are on the road, stock your car with healthy snacks and lots of water.
- Make sure you plan several stops each day for a little walk and a stretch.
- Think ahead about your vacation eating. For example, bring your own snacks; make a commitment to pass up rich desserts and have only one alcoholic drink a day.
- In a foreign country, try new foods but share them with a partner for portion control.
- Walk anywhere you can; restaurants, museums, etc. This will help to balance extra calories on your trip.

Entertaining (Away from Home or at Home)

Now that you understand how low fat cooking techniques contribute to permanent weight loss and overall good health, entertaining your friends is a wonderful way to introduce them to tasty new dishes. When you serve your friends low fat food, you are letting them know you care as much about their health as you do about your own.

- We suggest you delight your guests with your new *Fat Chance* recipes or your own recipes.

148

- Focus attention on the company and ambiance rather than just the food.
- Ask your guests to bring a dish that's low in fat and delicious. This is fun, educational and less stress on the hostess.
- Plan your drinks for those who drink alcohol and those who don't. Examples: cranberry juice and club soda with an orange slice, and a wine and soda cooler.
- Dress up your dishes with fresh flowers or herb sprigs, slices of fruit, berries, etc.
- If it's summer, plan some outdoor activities to go along with your entertaining, such as croquet, volleyball, Ping-Pong, etc. In winter, have some board games ready. In other words, plan activities so that eating is not the only thing to do.

> **The individuals who are most successful in achieving permanent weight loss are those who keep at it, in spite of occasional lapses.**

149

Many scientific studies have monitored the progress (or lack thereof) of people who are trying to lose weight. These studies show that one basic difference between success and failure in weight-loss programs is mainly due to the right or wrong kind of stimuli. That is why we have placed so much emphasis on building good food habits, avoiding tempting situations and having a supply of low fat snacks around at all times. The idea is to do everything possible to reinforce your good eating habits, and to do as much as possible to make bad eating habits inconvenient.

So, do eat out as often as you wish, but plan ahead of time what you are going to order, making sure that your food servings fit within the Food Pyramid. Be assertive, and ask the restaurant for what you want. And don't feel you have to finish everything on your plate just because it's there. Pay attention to your body, and learn to feel when you've had enough.

Of course, you won't change your old ways overnight, and there will be times when you slip up—we've all been through that. But another thing to keep in mind is that scientific studies show that the individuals who are most success-ful in achieving permanent weight loss are those who keep at it, in spite of occasional laps-es. In fact, there is a direct correlation between how long you stay with a weight-loss program and your degree of success.

> **If you have a fender-bender car accident, you don't stop driving do you?**

What makes us stay with a program? It's our confidence in what we're doing . . . our confidence that we will get the results we want. So let's begin to boost our confidence by changing our stimuli. From now on, you'll try to have healthy, low fat snacks around wherever you are, and you'll plan ahead when you eat away from home.

Our program is a day-to-day process, and each day will be different. Part of the process of replacing bad habits with good ones is to occasionally fail. If you have a fender-bender car accident, you don't stop driving do you? In fact, occa-sional failure is a normal part of getting where you want to go. But what will start to happen as you continue with our program is that you will gradually do the wrong thing *less* often and do the right thing *more* often. And that is a good definition of success.

> **"IT ISN'T THE HOURS ONE SPENDS AT THE TABLE THAT PUT ON THE AVOIR DUPOIS; IT'S THE SECONDS."**
> —*Jacob Brande*

STEP 30 — **Forgiveness, Patience and Taking Care of Yourself**

Forgiving Yourself

There will be some days when you really blow it—when you pig out on French fries or Fettucini Alfredo or a huge chocolate bar with guzillions of fat grams. What then? Well, you might be inclined to get depressed over what you've done and tell yourself that you have no will power, no ability to stick with it—so why not just give up and quit the program?

But if you think like that, you're missing the point. You haven't failed the test—you're in the middle of it.

Let's assume that you've been following our program for a week and that you've been able to reduce your fat intake while still enjoying tasty meals. Then, at the end of the week you succumb and eat a lot of fatty, high calorie food. In perspective, what have you done? You've had one bad day and six good ones. Not bad, especially for a beginner! Good enough for you to pat yourself on the back and say, "Pretty good job, so far."

And, in fact, you haven't failed at all. Occasional splurges are okay, and a part of our program is learning to be okay with this.

Patience

The second test is the test of patience. Let's assume you have been following our program (more or less—mostly more) for two months, but you haven't noticed much in the way of weight loss. Do you remember why? Way back in Step 3 we discussed your body's *set point*—how your body resists change for a while, even though you are consuming fewer calories, until the set point is overcome and you begin losing weight. And in Step 4 we talked about how muscle tissue is more dense than fat tissue—for example,

Occasional splurges are okay, and a part of our program is learning to be okay with this.

one pound of muscle takes up only ⅓ the space of a pound of body fat. So you will first start to lose *inches* rather than *pounds* as your body loses fat weight and gains muscle weight.

So don't weigh yourself. Instead, see if your clothes are starting to feel a bit looser.

But most important, realize that you didn't gain your weight overnight—it probably took years for it to accumulate, and it will take some time to reverse the process. Among those who have been successful at reaching their weight-loss goals, most took at least six months and some took up to two years.

Studies have also shown a beneficial side effect of patience is that the longer you stay with a weight-loss program, the greater your chances for eventual success. For example, persons who stayed on the program for three months were much more likely to continue on and succeed than those who quit after a single month. So each day you continue with it, the more likely it is you will succeed. Like everything else in life, you have to do it day-by-day, and Practice! Practice! Practice!

152

Taking Care of Yourself

If you have a family (even if your spouse may be helpful, considerate and emancipated), it's a pretty good bet that a lot of your time at home is spent caring for everyone else's needs before your own. Or, if you're a working woman, by the time you get home, clean the house, take an evening class, get your clothes ready, etc., there isn't much time to think about your own nutrition—so you gobble down whatever's handy.

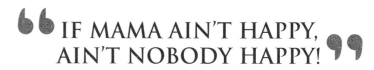

"IF MAMA AIN'T HAPPY, AIN'T NOBODY HAPPY!"

–Unknown

And this is a very common problem: Most of us are so busy doing other things that we don't allow ourselves enough time to make good food choices—for ourselves or for other family members.

There are no magic solutions for this: it's simply a matter of giving your personal nutrition a high priority. Here are some suggestions to help you get into the habit of making more time for yourself so that you can make good food choices:

- Plan for one prepackaged meal per week with your fresh vegetables.
- Do you have teenagers? Let them prepare one meal per week.
- Ask your spouse to prepare at least one meal per week.
- When you prepare a starch dish, make twice as much as you need, and use the starch again the next night. For example, make baked potatoes and for the next night, sauté them with onions.
- Try to arrange with a friend to share meal preparation. For example, you might cook for both families on Mondays and she'll do the same on Wednesdays.

153

Allow yourself some time each day . . . even if just a few minutes . . . to think about your food requirements for that day. Have there been changes in your schedule? Do you have any luncheon or dinner engagements planned? Are you taking the kids to the school fair (hot dogs, cupcakes, ice cream)? Do you have a long drive scheduled? Will you be entertaining friends?

Be prepared. Try to get into the habit of thinking about your own food needs—preferably ahead of time—for whatever events the day brings.

Co-dependency has been a big topic for the last several years, relating to alcoholics and their caretakers. But co-dependency spills over to the nonalcoholic household also. What is co-dependency? A clinical definition would be: "An emotional, psychological and behavioral condition that develops as a result of an individual's prolonged exposure to, and practice of, a set of oppressive rules; rules which prevent the open expression of feeling as well as the direct discussion of personal and interpersonal problems." In other words, you feel stuck in a situation that you can't talk about and that you can't seem to get out of.

Most women from 50 to 80 years old are caretakers. They were raised in an era when men were regarded as supreme and women were lucky to have a roof over their heads and "should know their place." Younger women feel more equal and responsible for all parts of their lives, which is a much healthier attitude.

How does this relate to health and eating? If you are always taking care of everyone else's needs, your own needs do not get met. If everyone else's schedule is more important than your own, you will never have time to exercise, and you will not make good food choices for yourself.

So a part of our program is to emphasize that *you* are responsible for your life, for your exercise and for your eating, and that *you* must make the time to take care of yourself! No fair blaming it on anyone else.

> **You are responsible for your life, for your exercise and for your eating, and *you* must make the time to take care of yourself!**

We've mentioned three things of great importance in this step. They're not tangible things; they're all about attitude, how you think about what you're doing.

Can you accept that occasional eating lapses are okay and remain determined to stay with this program in spite of them?

Can you be patient while your body is doing the things it needs to do before you start losing weight?

Can you give your own health needs a high priority? In short, can you take care of yourself?

Just as the *Little Engine That Could* said, "I think I can! I think I can! I think I can!" We know you can too!

154

Annette: This is a very important rule, Joan, and you know how I love rules.

Joan: Me too. So what's this 80-20 stuff?

Annette: Well, you know it's important to eat right and get good exercise exactly 80 percent of the days in each week.

Joan: 80 percent? Of seven days? But, Annette, that comes out to . . . let's see . . . that comes out to 5.6 days.

Annette: Right, 5.6 days per week.

Joan: Are you trying to tell our readers to eat right and get good exercise 5.6 days per week? Not 5.5 days? It has to be 5.6 days?

Annette: What's wrong with that?

Joan: Come on, Annette. How are we supposed to figure 5.6 days?

Annette: Relax, Joan, I'm just having a little fun.

Joan: Okay, I can go for some fun. So is there an 80-20 rule?

Annette: It's really a non-rule.

Joan: What do you mean?

Annette: Well, our readers deserve a break. There are enough rules around already.

Joan: Go on.

Annette: So our 80-20 rule is a non-rule. All it means is that we don't have to be perfect. We can give ourselves permission to slack off some of the time.

Joan: Like 20 percent of the time?

Annette: Something like that.

155

Joan: That sounds good to me. It's like discipline without deprivation.

Annette: Exactly. Just make sure you follow the rule.

Joan: The non-rule.

Annette: Right.

Joan: Well, thanks for the non-rule, Annette. I'm off to Baskin Robbins.

Annette: Wait for me!

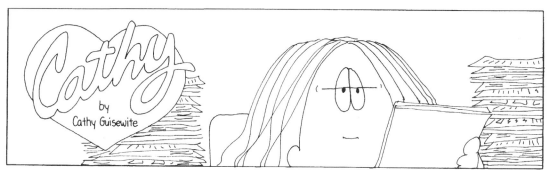

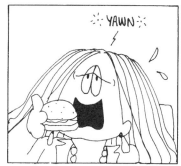

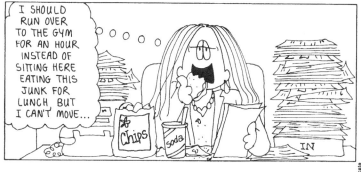

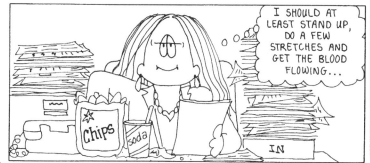

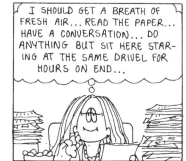

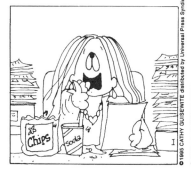

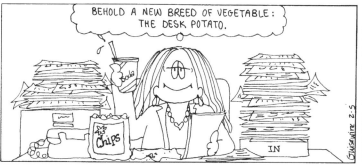

PART SEVEN

Can Fitness Be Fun?

STEP 32 — Why Exercise?

Drive-through restaurants, banks, dry cleaners and, in some areas, even drive-through wedding chapels. Inside our cars—power steering, power windows and power mirrors (in some models, even power cupholders so you don't have to extend your arm in order to pick up your drink). In our stores, escalators and powered doors that open and close themselves. In our homes, garage door openers and TV/stereo remotes.

In our modern society we have no time to waste, nor unnecessary energy to expend, so we have learned to make things as convenient as possible. But look at some of the elderly, or even the middle-aged people around you. First thing you notice is that many are overweight. Then you may notice that some are moving stiffly and awkwardly, as though their muscles and ligaments and bones aren't working well together. Yet many of them are not suffering from any specific disease—they are suffering from disuse.

Beginning in middle-age years, or perhaps even before, people gradually live a more sedentary life, which results in a gradual wasting away of muscle tissue, flexible joints and strong bones. This, in turn, becomes reason for doing even less, physically. A vicious circle emerges—less activity, weight gain, physical deterioration, even less activity, more weight gain, more deterioration.

157

Our bodies are made to move. When we don't use our muscles, we lose them.

But this scenario isn't a necessary part of aging. When you visit Europe, Asia or South America you don't see the obesity that is so prevalent in America, and older people often seem fit and vigorous. Why? A key factor is that even in other modern economies people are more physically active. There are fewer cars per person, so people walk and ride bikes more often. In addition to large-scale farming, many people still tend their own gardens.

Our prosperity in the United States has given us the option of being more and more sedentary, and if we don't do something about it, we will increasingly be left with poor health and shortened lives.

Our bodies are made to move. When we don't use them, they start falling apart, both inside and out. The resulting gradual weight gain and muscle loss is the catalyst for many adverse changes, including:

- Declining strength, flexibility and energy
- Less aerobic capacity
- Increasing bone weakness
- Decreasing circulation
- Decreased immune system activity—increased risk of disease
- Premature aged appearance

Back in Step 1, we explained in detail the connection between good nutrition and exercise in order to be *fit*. This is so important it bears repeating here.

What is fitness? It is the state, resulting from good nutrition and adequate exercise, that gives you the highest vitality, optimum body weight (for your particular body) and greatest resistance to disease and deterioration. Remember, when you reach a reasonable level of fitness, weight loss is an automatic side effect. Here's how it all fits together.

Permanent weight loss is a result of fitness.

1. **You will lose weight permanently only as you become more fit.**
2. **You will become more fit only by gaining more muscle, which burns more fat.**
3. **The only way to gain more muscle and burn more fat is through proper exercise, combined with healthy, low fat eating.**

So, in addition to being necessary for the maintenance of good health, exercise is also a necessary part of permanent weight reduction.

Exercise has a multiplier effect on weight reduction. For example, 20–30 minutes of aerobic exercise will raise your metabolism for several hours so that your body will continue to burn off additional fat from that relatively short exercise period. And even mild exercise, such as a stroll after a meal, will speed up the burning of calories so that less of them go into fat storage.

In addition to frightening you into exercising, we want to emphasize the positive as well. It is an absolutely wonderful feeling to be fit. When you are fit you feel more energetic, more confident, more at ease, happier, more sure of yourself—and in general, more alive. You'll have better skin tone, firmer muscles, fewer bulges—and all the overly tight clothes that you've saved (just in case) will fit once again. It's a great feeling! And once you start to get it, you won't ever want to lose it.

So, you see, there are many reasons why you should begin a regular exercise program along with your low fat eating. What we want to do in this section of the book is to help you become more aware of your body and how to exercise it properly. We want it to be enjoyable, to show tangible, positive results, and to become so much a part of your normal routine that it will become almost unthinkable for you to stop.

159

> **THOSE WHO THINK THEY HAVE NOT TIME FOR BODILY EXERCISE WILL SOONER OR LATER HAVE TO FIND TIME FOR ILLNESS.**
> *—Edward Stanley, Earl of Derby, 1873*

Since you are embarking on a permanent weight-loss program that will involve exercise, it's prudent to make sure your physical condition is up to it before you begin. Almost everyone can and should exercise, but some physical conditions may limit the kind of exercise you do, or its intensity, or cause you to emphasize certain exercises over others. There are very few physical problems that will require you to avoid exercise altogether.

Some obvious conditions that can limit your exercise program are problems connected with your heart and blood pressure, bone or joint limitations, or a tendency toward dizziness. It's important to remember that being active, even if it's only a little bit, will help you achieve better health. *If you believe you have any condition that may limit your exercise program, please consult your physician before beginning. If you are reasonably sure that your present health will not be an impediment, then begin–slowly and gradually.* Never take giant leaps forward in intensity or duration.

160

How Fat Are You?

Have you ever seen those tables, compiled years ago by insurance companies, that show *correct* weight for a given height? Sure you have, we all have. But how do they work for, say, body builders with a huge muscle mass? Or for distance runners, who are very lean? Do they work as well for Asians as for Europeans? How about the tall Masai in Africa, who might measure 6' 5" and weigh in at 110 pounds? Weight/height tables are only appropriate if you fit into the perfect average, which is unlikely.

So are you really overweight? For that matter, what's *overweight?* In fact, the term *overweight* is meaningless. What we should be saying is *overfat.* The real measure of fitness–the physical condition of your body–depends on several factors, including strength, flexibility, aerobic capacity and the amount of body fat present. It's important to keep the amount of body fat within a given range for several reasons. Body fat is storage; it's fuel for a future emergency. Other than a small amount of fat that the body actually needs in order to function, body fat isn't doing anything—it's just sitting there. We say that body fat is *metabolically inactive*.

Fat is metabolically inactive.

In contrast, your muscles, bones, organs, nervous tissue and skin are all working constantly to keep everything shipshape. We say that they are metabolically active.

Let's play the devil's advocate for a moment, and say, "So what? Why not let the body fat sit there—it's not hurting anyone, is it?"

Well, it's making us look plump and saggy, for a start, and causing excess

Muscles, bones, organs, nervous tissue and skin are metabolically active.

strain on our skeletal system to keep everything in its proper place. But there are several biological reasons why excess body fat isn't good for us. Studies have shown that too much body fat leads to heart disease, diabetes, hypertension and cancer. Furthermore, research has shown that body fat accumulates toxins—poisonous stuff that has been ingested or inhaled—which can, over a period of time, also increase our risk of disease.

161

But the presence of a high percentage of body fat is not, itself, the main problem. A high percentage of body fat is the side effect of loss of fitness, of loss of lean body mass. It is this loss which is so detrimental to good health. When we lose body fitness, we are decreasing the metabolically active part of our body and increasing the inactive part—the body fat that just sits there. Remember, when we lose muscle mass, we have less ability to burn off body fat. And so the downward spiral progresses: loss of lean body mass; less ability to burn off fat; more weight gain, and on and on.

So what we've been saying since the beginning of this book is that permanent weight loss and good health depend on fitness, and fitness depends on good nutrition and proper exercise.

Okay, by now we all agree we need to be *fit*. And we know that one way to measure fitness is to determine our total percentage of body fat. So there are two questions we need to answer: **1.** What is the optimum percentage of body fat for *you*? **2.** How can you determine *your* percentage of body fat?

Unlike the height vs. weight tables, which apply only to an average few, standards for percentage of body fat are pretty much universal. While some ethnic groups may have a somewhat lower or higher optimum standard, the ranges of body fat for optimal health apply to just about everyone. There are different standards for women and men, however, since men genetically have a lower percentage of body fat than do women.

Here are the ranges for percentage of body fat.

162

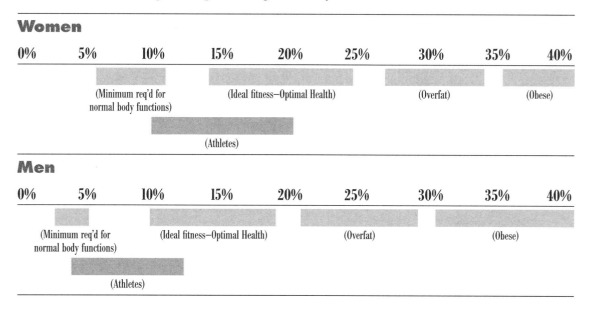

So for women, the optimal healthy range for body fat is 15–25%; for men it is 10–18%.

> ❝ BICYCLING AT 10 MILES PER HOUR
> USES THE EQUIVALENT IN FOOD ENERGY
> OF 1.4 OUNCES OF GASOLINE.
> THAT MEANS THAT THE HUMAN
> BODY GETS ABOUT 914 MILES PER GALLON. ❞
>
> *–Unknown*

Ways of Measuring Body Fat

Excess body fat is stored mostly as *subcutaneous* fat—which simply means that it is under the skin. This excess fat isn't limited to one area of the body but is spread around. Some people have skinny arms and shoulders, but heavy thighs and legs. Others are more egg-shaped, with large waistlines. Recent research has shown that this latter type of body fat distribution, known as *male-type* fat distribution, has been closely linked to increased risk of cardiovascular disease, diabetes and some cancers. Although called male-type distribution, women can also have this type of fat distribution. The point here is that if you are heaviest around your middle it is even more important to get rid of your excess fat because it is a definite health risk.

163

At what level does belly fat stop being a nuisance and start becoming a real health risk? Here's a quick test. Measure your waist with a tape measure, then measure your hips, and divide the waist measurement by the hip measurement. So if your waist is, for example, 32" and your hips are 39", then $32 \div 39 = .82$.

For a woman, your waist/hip ratio should be .8 or less. If you are .9 or above, you're likely to be at risk. For a man, your waist/hip ratio should be .9 or less. If you reach 1.0 or higher, you're likely to be at risk also.

Interestingly, if you are within the safe waist/hip ratio and you then gain weight equally around the waist and hips (so that the ratio stays the same even though you weigh more) there is not nearly as much health risk as if you gain more around the waist than around the hips. So if you have a pear shape, at least you can have the consolation of knowing it's much safer than if you look like a melon.

There are five basic ways of measuring overall body fat, four of which are somewhat impractical: chemical analysis, CAT scanning, electrical resistance, buoyancy and skin fold. Chemical analysis is probably the most accurate but requires a doctor and a sample (ouch!). CAT scanning shows a fairly accurate picture of how much fat is in your body, but this is a very expensive hospital procedure (which isn't covered by insurance). Electrical resistance is based on the fact that body fat conducts very tiny amounts of electricity differently than other tissue. This requires a specialist and the test is not widely available. The buoyancy test is based on the theory that being lighter, body fat floats; and being heavier, bones, muscles and organs sink. That's why overfat people are good floaters. The trouble with this test is that individuals have different body densities regardless of how much body fat they have (some have bigger, heavier bones, etc.), plus whether you float or not depends a lot on how much air is in your lungs at the time. The above methods can give you a reasonable estimate of your body fat, but they are impractical compared to measuring your body fat with skin calipers.

The Skin Fold Test

As we mentioned above, most of your body fat is deposited under your skin—but not equally under all of your skin. To prove it, try this. Gently pinch the skin on the underside or outside of your forearm. Try to find the place where the skin feels thinnest. That thinnest spot is the thickness of your skin without body fat. Now try the same thing . . . say . . . at the side of your waist or thigh. Notice a difference? Is it thicker? That's because the waist and thighs are two of the body's favorite places for depositing fat.

By carefully measuring the thickness of skin folds at various locations on

164

your body, it's possible to get a pretty good reading of your overall percentage of body fat. Skin fold tests are usually available at health clinics, fitness centers, spas and by consulting with a certified, personal trainer. An instrument called a skin caliper is used to accurately measure the amount of fat attached to your skin, in various locations on your body. We recommend that you have this test done once every 3–4 months, as the definitive measure of your progress.

Back in Step 4 we recommended, with tongue-in-cheek, that you throw away your scale. That was because as you become more fit, you will lose body fat and gain more muscle, and as a result, you will lose inches before you start to lose pounds. And those lost inches are a much better indicator of progress than lost weight. When your body contains the optimum percentage of fat, then you will also be at your optimum weight. That's why the skin fold test is so helpful.

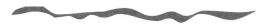

165

So the purpose of this step has been to acquaint you a bit more with your own body; first, to make sure you are in reasonable condition, without serious health problems, before you get started on an exercise program. And then to get you to think in terms of *overfat* rather than *overweight*–in terms of body composition rather than pounds.

Are you overfat? If you're like most Americans, the answer is yes. But now your goal will *not* be to lose a certain number of pounds, it will be to increase your fitness and reduce your overall percentage of body fat.

From the tables above, if you are a woman, your goal is to reduce your percentage of body fat to within the range of 15–25%, for optimum fitness. We're all together in this, you see. Now we all have the same goal. When *you* reach *your* goal, you may weigh 50 pounds more (or less) than either of us, but we will all be at an optimum percentage of body fat–we will all be fit.

STEP 34 — *So You Don't Wanna Look Like Arnold!*

Neither do we.

In Step 1, we mentioned that exercise is a necessary part of any permanent weight-loss program. In later steps, we'll describe why both aerobics and strength exercises are beneficial. One of the fears that some women have is that if they begin a fitness program that includes any kind of strength exercises, they will develop bulging, masculine muscles. Not true. Actually there are many men (and some women) who vigorously seek those kinds of muscles and still have a hard time getting them.

Large, defined muscles are not easy to develop. They are the result of very specialized, very strenuous weight-training programs. You have to really work at it. Unless you are doing one of these specialized programs, there is no chance of you developing bulging muscles (regardless of whether you're female or male).

If you want to make the cover of *Body Building,* our program's not for you. If you wouldn't mind looking slimmer, more streamlined, with tighter, smoother skin, and a more attractive shape, then we're talking the same language.

166

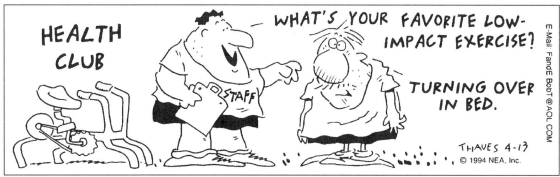

FRANK & ERNEST reprinted by permission of Newspaper Enterprise Association, Inc.

What do a body builder, a bicycle racer, a yogi and a ballerina have in common? Well, perhaps more than we might imagine, but one thing we know is that they all exercise. Yet, there is a vast difference in the effects of the exercise each of them is doing. Let's look at these effects by describing the various kinds of exercises that can be done.

Aerobic Exercise

The term *aerobic* means *in the presence of oxygen*. Aerobic exercise, or aerobics, is defined as continuous movement of the large muscle groups of the body so that their need for oxygen is increased. Examples of repetitive aerobics are dancing, brisk walking, jogging, skating, cycling and swimming. Examples of non-repetitive aerobics are activities with a lot of continuous movement, such as basketball and fast dancing. When the muscles need more oxygen, the lungs, heart and blood vessels respond by increasing the rate of oxygen delivery. The effect of this is to improve our cardiopulmonary system—to strengthen the lungs and heart, and to expand our blood vessels and keep them flexible. So the purpose of aerobic exercise is to improve our aerobic capacity, which means we are increasing our ability to take in, transport and utilize oxygen. When we increase our aerobic capacity, we become better fat burners.

167

Aerobic exercise also helps to:

- Decrease stress.
- Lower blood pressure.
- Stabilize blood sugar.
- Reduce unhealthy blood fats and increase healthy ones.
- Increase endurance.
- Enhance balance and coordination.
- Decrease appetite.

When we increase our aerobic capacity, we become better fat burners.

- Improve overall health and resistance to disease.
- Make bones stronger, preventing bone loss due to osteoporosis and reducing the likelihood of fractures.

Strength Exercise

Also called resistance training or weight lifting, this category of exercise forces muscles to work hard by introducing a resistance to their movement. Strength exercises can be done by using machines, free weights, elastic tubing, or by using the weight of your own body to create resistance (for example, pull-ups and push-ups). When you rely on your body alone for strength exercises, you force it to balance and stabilize itself instead of a machine stabilizing you. This will improve your coordination and balance.

168

> **Remember, the more muscle you have, the more fat you will burn.**

Although the purpose in strength training is not to develop bulging muscles, some increase in muscle mass is important because it will help us burn fat—remember, the more muscle you have, the more fat you will burn.

In addition to burning more fat, strength exercise is important because it also helps to:

- Make bones stronger.
- Maintain proper body posture and protect against lower back injury.
- Increase mobility and coordination.
- Reduce the possibility of muscle and tendon injuries.
- Improve balance and stability.
- Slow down the loss of function associated with aging.
- Enhance the ability to perform daily physical tasks without injury or discomfort.

When you begin strength training, some kind of professional assistance is usually necessary to help you understand the purpose of particular exercises. For example, a "wall sit" (squatting against a wall, holding your body in tension) is great for increasing muscle endurance for skiing, but it isn't recommended if you will be jogging, and it doesn't help remove fat from between your thighs. A certified personal trainer or a trainer at a fitness center can help you select exercises that are best for you.

Flexibility Exercise

Flexibility exercise, or stretching, is what allows us to move. We begin to lose this ability when we are physically inactive; when this happens, it's one of the warning signals that we are losing our fitness. What's so bad about becoming more stiff? Not only is it uncomfortable and inconvenient, it places more stress on our bones, muscles and joints, which can lead to severe injury. Yet for all its importance, stretching is the most ignored component of fitness routines.

Stretching should be a part of every workout. A comprehensive stretching routine performed after cooling down, when your muscles are most warm, will increase your range of motion and circulation, and decrease the risk of injury and muscle soreness/stiffness.

Stretching is also important because it:

- Helps maintain good body posture.
- Relieves tension and relaxes your body.
- Heightens your awareness of how to move and bend your body properly.

169

You need to achieve a balance.

Achieving a Balance

Returning for a moment to our body builder, bicycle racer, yogi and ballerina, what are the effects of their exercising? If the body builder only does strength exercises, the effect is very unbalanced—lots of muscle gain but little or no increased aerobic capacity or flexibility. Without flexibility, the body builder's greatly increased muscle mass will result in more stiffness and poor circulation.

> **"IF GOLF IS PLAYED FOR EXERCISE, HOW IS IT THE PLAYER WHO MANAGES TO GET THE LEAST OF IT WINS?"**
> *–Jacob Brande*

If the bicycle racer is not doing any additional exercise, she or he is getting a good aerobic workout, and a very strenuous use of certain leg and abdominal muscles (lower body), but the exercise is not balanced and there will be deterioration in the areas of the body not being used. The yogi is, of course, stretching everything along with some strengthening, but has a lack of aerobic exercise. Without supplemental exercises, his or her aerobic capacity will diminish along with all of its benefits.

170

That leaves the ballerina. She uses her body for resistance (strength), she must stretch in order to appear graceful, and the continuous dance routine trains her aerobically. The ballerina is a perfect example of incorporating all aspects of exercise into her fitness program. Another great aspect of the ballerina's program is that her exercises are *weight-bearing*—as she moves, she carries the weight of her body. The advantage of a weight-bearing exercise is that it places stress on your musculoskeletal system, which is one of the key factors in preventing osteoporosis.

In developing your own fitness program you need to achieve a balance between the work you place on your heart, your muscles and your body's frame. You will need to combine moderate, rhythmic movements, intense rapid movements, soft, relaxing movements and static, balancing movements. In other words, aerobic, strength and flexibility exercises need to be a part of your routine.

Cross-Training

Cross-training means doing a variety of different exercises as your fitness routine. Triathletes are examples of people who cross-train. They swim, bike and run, and probably do weight training as well. Cross-training doesn't have to be on the level of triathlons. It can be as simple as walking one day, playing tennis for the next workout, and using a rowing machine later in the week.

Cross-training goes beyond the example of the ballerina. It offers the advantages of working many different sets of muscles. Not only is this excellent for maintaining overall good health—remember that the more muscles you use, the more fat you burn—cross-training also decreases the chances of injury because you allow certain muscle groups to rest when you alternate activities. Also, chances are you'll be less bored if you have a variety of exercises in your fitness program.

And finally, doing only one kind of exercise increases some aspects of body fitness, but decreases others. For example, doing only aerobics can actually lessen the ability of muscles to perform strength tasks; and doing only strength exercises decreases the body's endurance. This makes it doubly important to have a variety of exercises in your fitness program.

So there you have it—variety and balance, which will result in less injury, less boredom, more fat burning and overall good health. We recommend cross-training highly!

171

Determining Your Level of Exertion

Have you heard about *target* heart rate? It's a term that is becoming increasingly well known. But what's the big deal? What is a *target* heart rate? Why bother trying to maintain your heartbeat at that rate? And how do you determine what *your* target rate is?

Well, your heart beats in response to how much oxygen-rich blood your body needs. When you are resting and relaxed, your heart beats relatively slowly and pumps relatively gently. The rate at which your heart beats when you are resting is called, aptly enough, its *resting rate*. When you are exercising, your muscles need more oxygen, and your heart responds by beating more quickly and strongly. If the intensity of your exercise continues to increase, your heart will reach a point where it's going flat out—it can't increase its pumping anymore. That point is called your *maximum rate*.

Your maximum heart rate temporarily gives you maximum body strength and speed, but it's like the family car. If you could find a place to legally do it and you drove your car at its flat-out top speed, you'd cover a lot of ground pretty fast, but you'd be placing a great deal of strain on the car, and wear and tear would result—possibly even a breakdown.

Same with your body. So unless you are an athlete-in-training, and are under professional supervision, you don't want to subject your body to the strain of exercising at your absolute, maximum capacity.

Now we said previously that increasing fitness depends on you doing more physical exertion than you've already been doing. That means you will need to get your heart beating faster than its resting rate when you exercise—that you will need to do aerobic exercise at an exertion level somewhere between your heart's *resting rate* and its *maximum rate*.

Over the years, fitness research has shown that there is a level of continuous exertion that achieves a very high rate of burning up calories, significantly

172

improves fitness—and is safe! Because the rate your heart is beating is the best indicator of overall bodily exertion, this efficient and safe level of exertion is called the *target range*—and it is measured by how many beats per minutes your heart is doing.

In order to do aerobic exercise at the most efficient level, safely, you need to keep your heart rate within the target range. Now there are many charts and tables and formulas that describe how to determine *your* target range. The trouble is, we are all individuals, and figuring what is right for you from these generalized formulas doesn't always work. Besides, some of them are complicated and bothersome to compute.

So, staying with our philosophy of keeping it simple, we'll forego all the formulas and give you three easy ways to help determine whether or not you are exercising within your target range.

The Golden Rule when learning how to pace yourself is: *listen to your body.*

173

1) The Talk Test

Okay. You and your exercise buddy are working on adjacent rowing machines at a fitness center. Five minutes into it, your buddy asks if you'd like to have lunch together after you've finished. You turn your head to reply, but the only thing that comes out of your mouth are the loud and rapid pantings of your breath. Guess what? You have gone beyond your target range. Ease off, and *find a level of exertion where you may be breathing hard but you can still speak easily.*

2) Perceived Exertion

The Golden Rule when learning how to pace yourself is: *listen to your body.* Perceived exertion is your own assessment of how hard you are exercising. We can put it in relative terms—for example:

Very Easy
Fairly Easy
Moderate
Hard
Very Hard
Very, Very Hard

When you're doing aerobics, try to work at a level of exertion that feels *moderate to hard*. Remember that what felt one way yesterday may feel differently tomorrow, so as you exercise, pay attention to what is happening NOW.

3) If You'd Like a Number

If you're more comfortable having an actual number for your target heart rate, then count your pulse (we count the pulses over 10 seconds and multiply by 6) while you're exercising at a level that feels moderate to hard. You may have to temporarily stop to do this, in order to feel your pulse clearly. In this manner, count your pulse several times during your exercise period and take the lowest and highest count you get as your target range.

Do this over a period of several days, and again, take your lowest and highest pulse counts as your target range.

Are you curious as to what average target rates are? Okay, if you're in your 30s, your likely target range might be around 125–150 beats per minute. If, for example, you're in your 50s, your target range might be around 110–135 beats per minute. (Your heart's ability to beat rapidly does decline with age.) And remember, these numbers are just to satisfy your curiosity—don't use them to judge *your* target range. Your range is determined by how *you* feel.

> **Try to work at a level of exertion that feels moderate to hard.**

174

Continuous and Interval Aerobics

As we have said earlier, the purpose of aerobics is to increase the capacity of your body's cardiopulmonary system—your lungs, heart and arteries. This enables you to deliver larger amounts of oxygen-rich blood to your muscles. This, in turn, improves your endurance and overall level of fitness, which enables you to burn more fat. Within the category of aerobics there are two forms: continuous and interval aerobics. With continuous aerobics, you exercise at the same pace for a minimum of 20 minutes. With interval aerobics, you alternately speed up and slow down during your exercise period.

While continuous aerobic exercise is certainly beneficial to permanent weight loss, interval aerobic exercise is even more so. Interval exercise makes your body more fit in the fastest, most efficient way. Because of this, your ability to burn excess body fat increases at the fastest rate, and you can see the effects of our program sooner.

Another term for interval aerobic exercise is *wind sprints*. Now don't let this term scare you off. It doesn't mean running at a very high speed until you are out of breath and puffing horribly.

What it means is that while doing your aerobic exercise, you occasionally go a bit faster than is comfortable—say for half a minute or a minute—and then return to your regular pace. If your aerobic exercise is walking, you might walk faster or even break into a jog for a short while. The same applies to whatever aerobic exercise you're doing; just do it a little faster and let yourself get just a bit out of breath, and then return to your normal pace, breathing comfortably before starting another interval.

With interval exercise, you'll become fitter faster, and you'll probably discover that it's actually fun to do.

175

STEP 37 — **Developing Your Own Routine**

How Much to Do?

Let's say your daily routine includes housecleaning, gardening, various errands and, perhaps, an evening stroll. While these tasks certainly include physical work, for our purposes, the question is: are your routine activities enough to bring you to a state of fitness and weight loss? If you're like most of us, probably not. Can you improve by doing just a bit more? For example, adding a 1-hour bike ride once a week? Well, that won't hurt. After all, any improvement is still an improvement.

But our goal isn't just a slight improvement—we're looking to achieve a high degree of fitness, with its side effects of permanent weight loss and overall good health. So how much do you have to do to achieve these benefits? Probably not as much as you think. There is a kind of minimum threshold with exercise and fitness. Maintain your exercise level at or above this threshold, and you get the desired results. Drop below the exercise threshold and you don't get the results.

Here are amounts of exercise we recommend: *The underlined figures indicate the bare minimum required to increase your fitness level.*

1. Aerobics: <u>4</u>–6 times per week, <u>20</u>–60 minutes each time
2. Strength Exercises: <u>2</u>–3 times per week, <u>6</u>–10 different exercises each time
3. Stretches: <u>3</u>–6 times per week (immediately following aerobics or strength exercises), <u>5</u> minutes each time

For aerobics, 4 times per week is the minimum; 5 times is very good, and 6 times per week is great! For strength exercises, more isn't better; stick to the 2 or 3 times per week. You can do stretches any time your muscles are warmed up—with stretches, it's pretty much the more the better, and the warmer your muscles are when you do them, the more effective your stretches will be.

Remember, it is important to take at least one day off per week to rest and rejuvenate your body—no physical exercise on this day.

176

Reps and Sets

A repetition, or "rep," is the number of times you repeat an exercise. If you do 12 squats, that's 12 reps. A "set" is the number of times you decide to repeat an exercise without a pause. So if your routine includes doing 12 squats without stopping, that's 1 set.

In our program we recommend that each set you do includes 12–15 repetitions of each exercise. A beginner may do only 1 set while an intermediate-level person might do 2 or 3.

Why 12-15 repetitions? In many strength exercises you have a choice of different resistance levels. At a fitness center, you can increase or decrease the weights on a machine. At home, you can do the milder or the more strenuous form of an exercise. In general, a small number of strenuous repetitions builds muscle bulk. A large number of less strenuous repetitions builds trim, shapely muscles. In this program, we are mostly interested in the latter.

Here's a good way of determining how strenuous an exercise should be. Adjust the resistance level so that the last 3 of your 12–15 repetitions feels hard to do—not painful, just to the point that you can't do the last 3 easily, with good form. That will be the right amount of effort to strengthen and trim your muscles. When the last 3 reps become easy, you'll know it's time to increase the weight.

Don't stop to rest within a set—finish the set and then rest a half minute or a minute between sets. If you are out of breath after a set, wait until you regain normal breathing before you begin the next set. But don't overly prolong the rest period, because you don't want your body to cool down between sets.

Developing Your Personal Routine

There are several aerobic activities to choose from (see Step 40). Between these and others that you can think of, choose one or more that you will be able to do at least four times each week. For ourselves, we like to do more than one for the

177

variety. Whatever helps you to keep doing it is the way to go. Don't feel committed to any particular choices—you can change at any time. You can do aerobics at home, at a fitness center, or a combination of the two. In terms of aerobics, it doesn't matter which exercises you do, as long as you are getting regular aerobic workouts.

For your strength and flexibility exercises, you can also choose to do them all at home, all at a fitness center, or a combination of the two.

If you choose to do them at home, here are two recommended routines.

At Home: Workout 1 (The following exercises are described in Step 41. Do one or two sets of each of the following, 2-3 times per week. Remember to warm up before you start, and cool down and stretch when you are finished.)

- Squats
- Stationary lunges
- Calf raises
- Seated rowing
- Dumbbell presses
- Prone lateral raises
- Bicep curls
- Dips
- Abdominal exercises

At Home: Workout 2 (One or two sets of each of the following, 2-3 times per week.)

- Step-ups
- Walking lunges
- Bridges
- Bent-over rowing
- Push-ups

178

- Prone lateral raises
- Bicep curls
- Tricep kickbacks
- Abdominal exercises

To make sure you are doing these correctly and safely, we suggest you use the services of a certified trainer to get you started.

There are many options to choose from at a fitness center. All fitness centers have trainers to help you develop a personal routine, based on your present condition, your goals and the available equipment. Be sure to seek the help of one of these specialists if you choose to exercise at a fitness center.

> **It doesn't matter which exercises you do, as long as you are getting regular aerobic workouts.**

Keeping Records

It's not necessary to keep elaborate records of your exercise program, but you'll find that two simple kinds of recordkeeping will help keep you on track. For aerobics, you need only keep a log of the number of minutes spent on aerobics each week. Your record can look like the following, or any variation of it you choose.

179

Aerobics Log, Week of _____

	SUNDAY	MONDAY	TUESDAY	WEDNESDAY	THURSDAY	FRIDAY	SATURDAY
Type of activity							
No. of minutes							

Total no. of workouts this week _____

Average no. of minutes per workout this week _____

Congratulations! Another week of good workouts!

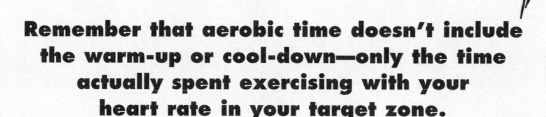

Remember that aerobic time doesn't include the warm-up or cool-down—only the time actually spent exercising with your heart rate in your target zone.

It's helpful to do this in a calendar style so you can see how you are spacing your exercise. Theoretically, if you do aerobics only four times each week, on three consecutive days (including twice on one day), you could have a period of four days with no aerobic exercise. It's best to space it out as evenly as you can during the week, so there are no lapses longer than two days.

For keeping records of strength exercises, you'll find that each fitness center has it own form of log that will track the exercises you do, the weight you use for each, and the number of repetitions. For keeping records of this at home, you can use the chart on the following page or any variation of it.

Should Exercises Be Done in Any Order?

In general, work larger muscle groups first (legs, back, chest). Working your large muscle groups increases blood circulation throughout the body. Also, if you work small muscles first, they will fatigue more quickly without that increased circulation, and this will affect your form when you start to work your larger muscles.

How about Seasons of the Year?

Try not to let bad weather interrupt your fitness routine. Work around it. It's important to maintain a continuous, year-round exercise program. Remember that your body's level of fitness decreases quickly when you are sedentary and it takes much longer to regain that lost fitness when you begin exercising again.

Have you ever exercised on a hot day and just felt wilted afterwards? Too much heat or cold can definitely make your workout grueling. During the summer months, try to exercise when the heat is at a minimum—early morning or

180

Strength Training Log

EXERCISE	DATE	SET	1	2	3	1	2	3	1	2	3	1	2	3	1	2	3	1	2	3	1	2	3	1	2	3	1	2	3	1	2	3
		Weight																														
		Reps																														
		Weight																														
		Reps																														
		Weight																														
		Reps																														
		Weight																														
		Reps																														
		Weight																														
		Reps																														
		Weight																														
		Reps																														
		Weight																														
		Reps																														
		Weight																														
		Reps																														
		Weight																														
		Reps																														
		Weight																														
		Reps																														
		Weight																														
		Reps																														
		Weight																														
		Reps																														
		Weight																														
		Reps																														
		Weight																														
		Reps																														

late evening. If you are outside, wear plenty of sunscreen; if you are inside, try to have a fan directed toward you. Remember to drink plenty of water. When the winter months arrive, make sure you dress in layers so that you can peel off your clothes as you get warmer. Protect your air passages from very cold air with a scarf, especially if you are doing high intensity exercise which will deepen your breathing.

Exercise Is Individual

If Jane Fonda can do it, I can too! Wrong! Many people push themselves too fast because they want to be like someone else. Remember that exercise is individual. Your own capacity is dependent on many variables, including age, genetic endowment, living habits and general health. Always focus on your own improvement rather than comparing yourself to someone else.

Exercise and Age

Age is no barrier to fitness. Everyone—even the elderly—do become more fit through exercise. It may take older persons a while longer to reach a good level of fitness, but exercise benefits everyone, *without exception*.

Too Much Too Soon

You've been sedentary for the last couple of years. You want to change this, so you embark on an exercise plan suited for an athlete who's going to the Olympics. A week later you feel like a veteran who barely survived the war. Sound familiar? This is the saga of many who want to lose weight quickly and know they have to exercise in order to do it. But doing too much, too soon will only backfire on you. Not only does it increase your risk of injury, it leaves you feeling burnt out. An exercise program *must begin slowly*, and *gradually progress in intensity, frequency and duration*. You should not increase your activity by more than 10% per week. For example, if you start by walking 20 minutes three

182

times a week, and you want to increase your walking time, you should only add 2 minutes to each day's walk the following week. And about 2½ minutes the next week, and so on.

Clothing and Accessories

The first items you need to consider when trying to make exercise comfortable are your shoes and clothing. Your shoes should provide support, stability and comfort, and should be designed for the exercise you are doing (for example, you wouldn't wear tennis shoes to go running). Your clothes should not bind or constrict your movement. It's best to wear outfits made of breathable fabric. It is also important to wear undergarments that are comfortable and supportive. You can find appropriate workout clothing in sports stores, department stores and athletic shoe stores.

The Time of Day

Exercise increases your metabolism and keeps it higher for several hours after you have stopped. Combined with moderate activity for the remainder of the day, the effect of exercising early is to burn off more calories than if you had exercised later in the day. There is also a second benefit of early exercise: as the day progresses, you are usually more involved with people and events, and it's easy to forego the exercise. If it is done early in the day, you've got it behind you before projects and chores close in on you.

183

Exercise and Eating

You've been busy all day and haven't had time to eat. Now it's time to go to the gym. You start your regular routine but after a few minutes you're worn out and can't understand why you don't have any energy. When this happens, you should ask yourself, "Can a car go very far without any gas?" We are built the same way. Our bodies need fuel and if they don't get some they're not going to work as well. This doesn't mean you have to eat a large meal just before exercising. But you should have a moderate amount of food sometime in the two-hour period before exercising. You might try keeping something in your car to munch on as you head for the gym, or for after your workout on the way home.

Exercise and Warm-ups

The purpose of a warm-up is to gradually prepare your body for more vigorous exercise by slowly raising muscular temperature and increasing blood flow to the working muscles. The best way to warm up is to use your large muscle groups (legs, buttocks) in activities like walking, exercycling or rowing. For example, if your aerobics exercise is to be a 30-minute brisk walk, start with an easy walking pace for 5–10 minutes.

184

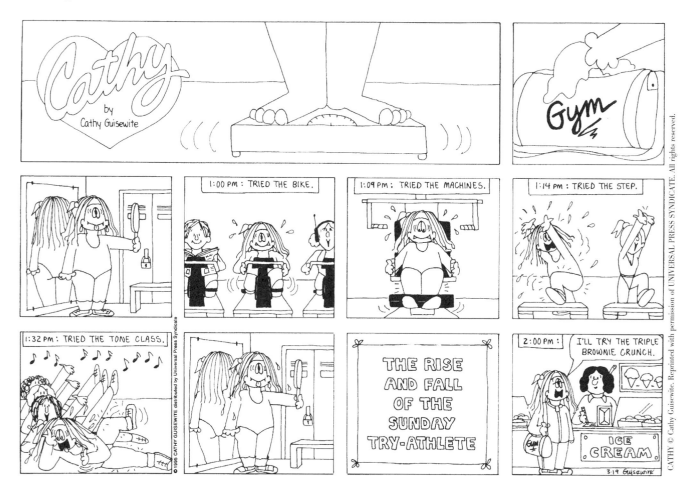

Always warm up before beginning your exercise routine. When you begin, remember that bodies don't like abrupt changes. Always start slowly and increase gradually.

Exercise and Cool-downs

A cool-down is the reverse of a warm-up—it is the gradual tapering off of activity. Its purpose is to allow the body to gradually return to normal circulation patterns. Aerobic activity increases blood flow to the lower extremities, and cooling down prevents blood from pooling in this area, away from the heart. Also, when you exert your muscles, some unwanted by-products are created. Cooling down gradually removes these elements from the muscles so your body can dispose of them.

For a cool-down, you can do your warm-up in reverse; for example, after your brisk walk, walk at a moderate pace and gradually slow down over 5–10 minutes.

Horses and dogs need cool-downs after hard exercise—so do we.

Exercise and Breathing

It's good to continue breathing while you exercise. Seriously though, some people get in the habit of holding their breath during certain parts of a strength exercise. Don't do this. The way to breathe properly when exercising is to exhale as resistance is increased and inhale when you relax.

Your Competitive Spirit

If part of your exercise program includes competitive sports, fine—compete. Otherwise, forget about what everyone else is doing. Trying to compare who is ahead and who is behind on an exercise program won't work; each body is different; focus on your own program.

Pain and Gain

The key to proper exercise is to *stress* the body without *straining* it. When you

185

stress your body, you are pushing it slightly beyond what it is used to; when you push it farther, to the point of experiencing pain, you are setting yourself up for setbacks and possible injury. So let the masochists (and some professional athletes-in-training) deal with pain. For purposes of improving fitness, if you feel pain while exercising, ease off on your intensity, speed or whatever else is causing it. If that doesn't help, stop temporarily until the pain is gone. Exercise should not be painful; if it is, you are doing something wrong.

Speaking of pain, turn to the next step to see how you can avoid back pain by keeping good posture.

186

Not only exercise, but simply doing the daily chores can result in unnecessary back injury. Let's do our best to avoid the back problems that are often caused by two incorrect ways of moving: arm lifts and knee bends.

Arm Lifts

Try this. Stand upright with your arms at your sides. Now slowly begin raising both arms until they are raised high over your head. Do you feel your lower back arching as you raise your arms? If so, you are inviting back trouble. Now let's try it again—this time, correctly. Stand upright with your arms at your sides. Now tuck your buttocks in and tighten your abdominal muscles (abs). Another way of saying this is to rotate your lower pelvis forward. Can you feel your lower back flatten as you do this? Now relax again, and note the correct positions in the following illustration:

As you raise your arms, consciously tuck your buttocks in and tighten your abs. Don't let your back arch. Then, as you lower your arms again, slowly relax your buttocks and pelvis. This is the correct way to lift your arms and to do strength exercises involving arm lifting. Practice this several times until it starts to become habitual. The goal is for it to become automatic whenever you lift your arms.

187

Knee Bends

Try bending your knees and lowering yourself to a squatting position. Use a wall or any stable object for balance if necessary. When you are squatting, note the position of your knees. Are they over your ankles, toes or forward of your toes? Okay, that's enough—stand up again.

Most of us are used to squatting the wrong way, with our knees too far forward. This puts excessive strain on muscles and joints. The correct way to do knee bends is to extend your buttocks as far backward as you comfortably can as you squat, positioning your knees and most of your body weight over your feet. Note the correct positions in the following illustration:

Now let's try it. As you squat, extend your buttocks as far backward as you comfortably can to maintain an arch in your lower back. Keep your heels on the floor and your knees over your feet. It's okay to point your feet outward. This is the correct way to bend and pick up an object from the ground.

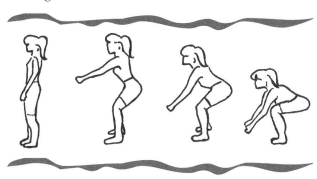

188

It will take a little time and practice to be able to bend and balance correctly. As with the arm lifts, the goal is to make it automatic, so that your weight shifts backward each time you bend your knees for any purpose.

Other Back-Saving Tips

- Never bend and twist your back at the same time—move your feet to turn your body.
- Keep objects close to your body when lifting or carrying.
- Stretch your legs often.
- If something is too heavy to lift comfortably, get help.
- When sitting, try to keep your knees lower than your hips.
- Don't let back braces or weight belts be a substitute for strong abs and buttocks muscles.
- Work your abs! Work your abs! Work your abs!

STEP 39 — **What about Your Tummy?**

"**S**it-and-twist," "Belly-buster," "Sidemaster"—these are some of the gadgets and devices we buy in our quest to have a slim and toned middle. It is an area of our body we are seldom happy with. But, unfortunately, many of us go about trying to get rid of our belly bulge in the wrong way. Traditional sit-ups, leg lifts and gadgets just won't do the trick.

In this step you'll learn how to do the most effective exercises for your abdominal muscles (and they're simple, too!), and you'll see why it is so important to have strong abs, which is what we call them for short.

But first you need to know that if you are carrying fat around your middle, the best way to get it off is with aerobic exercise, *not* stomach crunches. Abdominal exercises will strengthen your stomach muscles underneath the fat but they won't take the fat away. You need to burn fat off with aerobic exercise!

Vanity is not the only reason to strengthen our abs. They are perhaps the most important muscles of our body. They stabilize our torso, help our posture, protect our vital organs and support our lower back. Our abs are the core of our body's structural system and we need to keep them strong and balanced. The following routine will do just that—in the most efficient way.

189

Reverse Curl

a. Lie on your back with your knees bent and your feet flat on the floor (alternately, you can have your legs on a chair and your knees at right angles—see clam exercise, **c** and **d,** on next page).

b. Inhale deeply, allowing your middle to expand. Now slowly exhale and at the same time tilt your hips upward, pressing your back down onto the floor. Don't let your hips come off the floor.

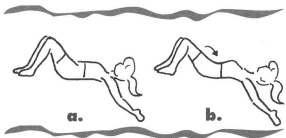

Contract your abdomen (pulling your belly button closer to your spine) while exhaling all of the air in your lungs. It's important to keep your belly flat and force all of the air out because this is what works the deepest layers of your abs. Then relax and breathe in. Repeat.

Clam

a. Lie on your back with your knees bent, and your feet flat on the floor about shoulder-width apart. Cup your hands under your head. **b.** Slowly raise your upper torso off the ground. Don't pull on your neck, keep it in line with your trunk by keeping your elbows back. Do the reverse curl procedure (as described above) simultaneously as you raise up. Exhale as you exert upward, inhale as you come down and relax. Alternately, you can cross your hands over your chest and you can have your legs on a chair with your knees at right angles (**c** and **d**).

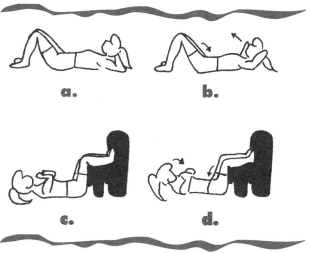

The reason this exercise is called a *clam* is because your belly button is the axis, much like a clam shell. During this exercise your upper and lower body are being squeezed upward while you try to keep your belly button close to the ground.

For a more advanced version of this exercise, keep your arms straight, outstretched above your head.

❝HE WHO DOESN'T MIND HIS BELLY ❞
WILL HARDLY MIND ANYTHING ELSE.
—*Samuel Johnson*

Slide-Ups

a. Lie on your back with your knees bent and your feet about shoulder-width apart. Cup your left hand under your head. Place your right hand across and onto the outer part of your left thigh. **b.** Keeping both hips on the ground, contract your abdomen and slide your right hand upward along your left thigh. Hold this for a count of five. Exhale as you contract and raise your hand, inhale as you come down and relax.

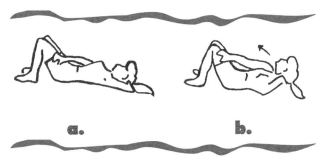

Repeat the mirror image of this, placing your left hand on your right thigh.

Reverse Trunk Twists

191

This is an advanced abdominal exercise for people with strong abs and no back problems.

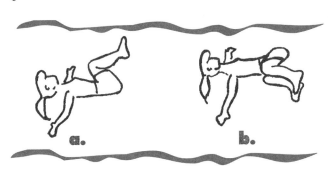

a. Lie on your back, arms out-stretched to the sides (your arms and body forming a letter "T"), palms on the floor, hips and knees bent at right angles. Keep your shoulders on the ground throughout the exercise. **b.** Keeping your knees together, slowly lower your legs to the right side of your body. Smoothly raise your legs back up to the starting position and then lower them on the other side. Repeat.

Abdominal exercises can be performed as often as four times per week, spread out over as many days as possible. Do each exercise slowly and smoothly. Begin with 5–10 repetitions of each exercise, and gradually work up to 25 or more.

> **When doing these or any other exercises, stop immediately if you should experience any unusual pain and consult a sports medicine practitioner to determine the source of the problem.**

192

Essentially, every exercise you do includes working your abs. Keep your tummy tucked in for whatever exercise you are doing. This goes for when you are standing, sitting, lying down or kneeling.

When lying down, don't secure your feet under a couch or other heavy object in order to make the exercise easier—this allows your hip flexors to take over the work of your abs.

So, throw away your gadgets and start working your abs the right way! And, remember, tummy rolls will disappear only with aerobic exercise!

STEP 40 — Aerobic Training: Your Fat-Burning Exercises

Machines at the Fitness Center

The advantage of a fitness center is having a large variety of equipment at your disposal. A disadvantage is that the equipment is not always available (someone else is using it or it's being repaired), and this is a problem if your time is limited. Some of the most popular aerobics machines are stationary bicycles, rowers, treadmills, stair steppers and cross-country skiing machines.

Stationary Bicycling *(Intensity level: moderate to high)*

This is probably one of the most simple and safe ways to get a good aerobic workout. A great feature of stationary bicycling is that you can read or watch your favorite TV show at the same time.

It's important to have the proper seat adjustment to keep your leg muscles in balance and to prevent injury. Your leg should be almost fully extended but not locked straight (your knee slightly bent) when it is at the lowest point of the pedaling circle. You should not have to move from side to side on the seat as you pedal; if you do, the bike seat is too high.

Recumbents are a variation of the upright stationary bicycle. These are ridden in a reclining position. In an upright position your torso weight is placed fully upon your buttocks, while in a reclining position your weight is distributed throughout your back, lower back and buttocks. Aerobically, there is no difference between the upright and recumbent bikes; it's just a matter of personal comfort.

Rowing *(Intensity level: high)*

Rowing is probably one of the best indoor exercises you can do, because it provides aerobic benefits while strengthening both the upper and lower body without impact or strain to muscles and joints.

To get into a smooth rhythm, push out with your legs, then pull with your

193

arms; when you are fully extended, release the pressure on your arms and let the gripping handle return, then curl your legs to return to the starting position. It helps to think, "legs - arms - arms - legs." Remember to sit up straight while rowing so you use your back and abdominal muscles properly.

Some rowing machines have TV screens which show your position compared to another boat. By entering the speed you want to row, you are setting the speed of the other boat, with which you will have to keep up. By displaying your position next to the other boat, the TV screen shows if you are keeping up with the pace you selected, if you are ahead or falling behind.

A common mistake in beginning with a rowing machine of this kind is to set the speed too high. Remember, this is a high-intensity exercise. It's common to see beginners with purple faces, huffing and puffing, and quitting after a few minutes. So start out slowly and see how it feels before you go to the Olympics rowing level.

Treadmill *(Intensity level: low to high, depending on speed and angle)*
Treadmills are a great choice for aerobics because of their range of intensity. They can work for the beginner or the elite runner. Many treadmills can be elevated to an upward angle to increase the required exertion. Treadmills are like moving sidewalks and it may be awkward to walk on them at first. Go ahead and hold onto the rail until you are comfortable with the movement. When you are comfortable, let your arms go and start swinging them by your side to work your upper body.

Stair Stepper *(Intensity level: moderate to high)*
Stair stepping machines, also known as stair climbers, are very popular in fitness centers and they do offer a great workout without the impact to your joints. A problem with stair climbers is the potential to position yourself incorrectly. To get the most out of this exercise, you should stand straight and only lightly hold on

to the bars for balance—don't lean forward as you hold on. With some practice you should be able to balance without holding onto the bars at all.

Some people use stair steppers at the highest level, locking their elbows and wrists on the bars and tiptoeing frantically on the steps. This takes the workload off of the legs and places a huge amount of strain on the tendons of the wrists and arms. So if you feel you cannot do the stair stepper without gripping the bars, skip this machine—at least until you can get some professional guidance on using it.

Cross-Country Ski Machine *(Intensity level: very high)*

Cross-country skiing machines use more muscles than most other aerobic machines. The movement is very strenuous, but because you glide instead of bounce, you do not impact your muscles and joints. The challenge with this exercise is that it requires balance and a lot of coordination. You may want to start by using your legs only and slowly integrate your arms as you feel comfortable.

It's easy to overdo it with this one, so start slowly and increase only gradually.

Exercise Riders *(Intensity level: moderate to high)*

Exercise riders are similar to cross-country ski machines in that they give a total body workout (without the need for coordination required by the ski machines). You ride these machines in a seated position and your lower body pumps while your upper body pulls. You can increase the intensity with height and handlebar adjustments, but the basic movement stays the same.

The important thing to remember when using this machine is proper posture. Always keep your abdominals tightened throughout the movement. If your abdominal muscles are weak and you find you cannot keep them contracted while working this machine, then don't use this machine until you are stronger. Also, emphasize pumping with your legs more than pulling with your upper body.

195

When used with the proper posture, exercise riders are a great way to burn fat and strengthen your muscles without any impact to your joints.

Fitness Machines at Home

Many of the machines you see at fitness centers are available for home use as well. These machines allow you the convenience of exercising at home and on your own schedule. Yet most people who buy home fitness machines stop using them after a short time. Here's how to avoid this.

With some types of products you can get away with buying a cheap version, but this is usually not the case with fitness machines. Cheap machines usually end up in the garage or closet, unused. Goodwill thrift stores are filled with cheap exercise machines whose owners got rid of them.

In general, the heavier and more expensive the machine, the better it is. Before buying one, try it out—not just for a few moments—but for the full amount of time you will be using it (for example, a minimum of 20 minutes). That's the only way to tell if some poorly designed feature will prove uncomfortable or unworkable for you. Remember, always try it before you buy it.

Before you buy a fitness machine, see if you can rearrange your furniture so that you can set aside a permanent place for the machine. If you have to drag it out and put it away after each use, chances are you'll stop pulling it out after a while.

Have a TV or stereo and a book rack nearby (here's where a TV "remote" really comes in handy). Having the phone reachable from the machine can save you lots of interruptions (or else turn the phone off while you are exercising).

You'll probably be more comfortable if your at-home aerobic room is cool, with good air ventilation. Make your aerobic exercise as convenient and comfortable as you can, and it will be more likely that you'll keep it up.

196

Examples of Other Aerobic Activities

Swimming *(Intensity level: moderate)*

Swimming is a wonderful workout if you are a competent swimmer. It's a time when you are in your own thoughts, your own world, moving through refreshing, calming water. It is an activity for the whole body—exercising the shoulders, arms, chest, back, trunk, hips and legs. The water's buoyancy allows the muscles and joints to work without impact, making swimming the most injury-free activity you can do. The smooth rhythmic motion of swimming both stretches and strengthens the body.

If you choose swimming as one of your frequent activities, we strongly recommend you protect your eyes with goggles, your hair with a cap and your skin with sunscreen if you're outdoors.

Other water activities like aqua aerobics, water polo or hydro-walking are great ways to get fit with little stress to the joints and ligaments.

Walking *(Intensity level: low to moderate)*

Walking is an aerobic exercise that is suited for almost everyone. We already have the equipment (our legs); it can be done just about anywhere; it is not high impact, so risk of injury is low; it does not require any special skill, and you can even walk in shopping malls when the weather is bad. (Window shopping doesn't count!)

If you're going to walk as an aerobic exercise, remember that easy strolling won't do it—you have to walk at a brisk enough pace to get your heart rate into your target range. (Remember *target range?* See Step 36 if you've forgotten.) You want to walk fast enough so that your exertion level feels moderate to hard, but not that you're so out of breath you can't talk. Here are the perceived exertion levels we mentioned in Step 36.

197

Very Easy
Fairly Easy
<u>**Moderate**</u>
<u>**Hard**</u>
Very Hard
Very, Very Hard

Wear the right kind of shoes. Choose a shoe which provides good padding, stability, traction and, especially, arch support. Try different shoes on in the store, practice walking in them at your target pace, and get the ones with the best fit.

Hiking *(Intensity level: moderate to high, depending on terrain)*
What's the difference between *walking* and *hiking?* For us, the difference is where you are. If you're walking on a paved path or sidewalk in town—that's walking. If you're on a trail that winds through the hills and goes up and down—that's hiking. Hiking is usually more intense than walking because you are constantly having to alter your movements to step over rocks, climb a hill, etc., and that takes more energy.

Hiking is an aerobic activity that is great for the whole family.

If you don't take unnecessary chances (leaping over a chasm, walking right up to the edge of a cliff), hiking is quite safe, and it is one of the most enjoyable of aerobic exercises—the view is constantly changing, and just being close to nature is rewarding. This is also an aerobic activity that is great for the whole family.

Jogging *(Intensity level: moderate to high)*
Jogging offers one of the fastest ways to get fit aerobically, and lose excess fat—but with it comes the possibility of injury to the joints, ligaments and muscles of the

198

lower body. Jogging is definitely an activity of personal choice; some love it and even get a "runner's high," while others find it jarring, uncomfortable and too intense.

If you are going to jog regularly, you need to have good shoes. To minimize the jarring to your body, try running on the softest ground that is available. A dirt track or a hard-packed sand beach is great. A black-top road is much easier to run on than a concrete sidewalk (when you've been jogging for a while, you'll begin to notice that some pavements are harder than others).

Always warm up by walking before you start to jog. If you have never jogged before, you should start off with aerobic walking. When walking briskly for 30 minutes feels easy, you are ready to add short jogs . . . up to 30 seconds. As you become more used to jogging, lengthen your jogs to about 100 yards (the length of a short city block). Do this three or four times during your 30-minute walk. Gradually, as your body gets more adept at jogging, you can increase the duration of your jogs until you are able to jog for most of the 30 minutes (always remembering to warm up and cool down with walking).

199

Aerobic Dance *(Intensity level: moderate to high)*

Aerobic dance routines are available on many videos, but many have poorly designed, high-impact routines with dangerous stretches. This results in many injuries. Whether on video or in a live group, make sure that the dance instructor has been certified and has up-to-date knowledge and skills.

Aerobic dance offers many factors which make exercising fun: music, creativity, camaraderie and variety. To begin, make sure you have good shoes and a safe, unobstructed area. If the aerobic dance routine doesn't include a warm-up and/or cool-down, then be sure to add your own.

There are many variations to aerobic dance: step aerobics, cardio funk, low impact aerobics and line

> **Aerobic dance offers many factors which make exercising fun: music, creativity, camaraderie and variety.**

dancing, just to name a few. They are all fun, but you must have good form, so if you are following a video (where you don't have a live instructor to give you feedback) pay close attention to the leader.

Ice and Roller Skating *(Intensity level: moderate to high)*

These are both very good, low impact aerobic exercises, which use almost all the muscle groups in your body. The gliding motion is especially helpful for slimming and tightening thighs. However, if you're just starting either of these, take it very easy at first; you'll be using your muscles in different ways than your body is used to, and it's easy to injure something or, at the very least, get quite sore.

Outdoor Rowing *(Intensity level: moderate to very high)*

As with the rowing machine, rowing a boat offers a smooth, non-jarring use of all muscle groups. It is particularly suitable for people who want to do an outdoor exercise but whose injuries prevent them from walking, cycling or other aerobic activities. In contrast to rowing, canoe and kayak paddling offer a less intense exercise, with more emphasis on arm and shoulder muscles.

Sports Activities

There are many popular activities, both in team sports and in individual sports, that are great fun and burn calories but which may not be *aerobic* because there is a lot of stopping and starting. The main criterion of aerobic exercise is that it be steady and continuous.

For example, singles tennis may keep you on the run most of the time while in doubles tennis, you spend a lot of time standing still. A 2-person team of volleyball will be continuously high intensity, but if you are 1 of 8 persons on a team, you'll spend a lot of time just watching. So whether your interest is soccer,

200

The main criterion of aerobic exercise is that it be steady and continuous.

fencing, Ping-Pong or downhill skiing, and you want to do these activities for the aerobic benefits, pay attention to whether or not you're keeping a steady pace.

If you'd like to compare the calorie-burning effects of different aerobic activities, here's a table that shows some of them. The table assumes that for each activity, you are performing the activity at the perceived exertion level of *moderate to hard*, as we have previously defined it.

Remember, it is more important to focus on choosing an activity you enjoy rather than focusing on how many calories you burn for a certain activity. What matters is that working your muscles makes you more fit.

ACTIVITY	Calories Burned over 30 Minutes of Exercise for Different Body Weights				
	120 LB.	140 LB.	160 LB.	180 LB.	200 LB.
Basketball	205	239	273	307	341
Bicycling	105	120	138	155	173
Canoeing	108	126	144	162	180
Dancing, Aerobic	252	294	336	378	420
Dancing, Ballroom	72	84	96	108	120
Fencing	144	168	192	216	240
Hiking	160	185	211	237	264
Jogging	180	210	240	270	300
Jumping Rope	235	273	313	352	391
Kayaking	90	105	120	135	150
Martial Arts	216	252	288	324	360
Ping-Pong	101	121	139	156	174
Rowing	210	245	279	314	349
Skating, Ice	162	189	216	243	270
Skating, Roller	198	231	264	297	330
Skiing, Cross-Country	108	126	144	162	180
Swimming	218	255	294	331	368
Tennis, Singles	162	189	216	243	270
Volleyball	144	168	192	216	240
Walking	140	170	195	219	244

201

Some Things to Remember

- Do a variety of aerobic activities at least 4 times per week for at least 20 minutes each time.
- Begin slowly and gradually progress in intensity, frequency and duration (no more than 10% increase per week).
- Exercise at an exertion level that feels moderate to hard, but not that you're so out of breath you can't talk (the exception to this is during the intense part of interval training).
- Wear the right kind of shoes and clothing.
- Always warm up and cool down.
- Incorporate interval training to help you get more fit!

202

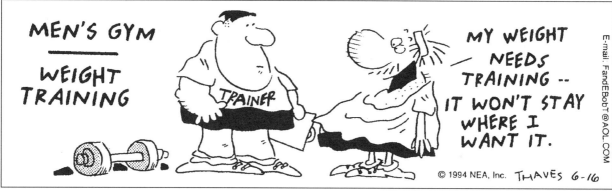

FRANK & ERNEST reprinted by permission of Newspaper Enterprise Association, Inc.

STEP 41 — Strength Training: Your Muscle-Toning Exercises

 A **Few Pieces of Necessary Equipment**

To do a well-rounded program of strength exercises at home, you will need a bit of inexpensive equipment and some props. The most basic equipment is a set of handheld weights called dumbbells. These are now available in all stores that carry sporting equipment. Alternate hand weights come in the form of weighted wristbands. Dumbbells have the advantage of being more convenient, but weighted bands can be used for both wrists and ankles.

For a beginner, we recommend you get two of each of the following weights: 1 lb., 2 lb., 3 lb., 5 lb., 8 lb. For those who have been doing strength exercises for some time, we recommend two of each of the following weights: 5 lb., 8 lb., 10 lb., 15 lb., 20 lb. If, for any reason, you can't get these small dumbbells, try using plastic water containers. You can fill them with sand, bird seed or buckshot to the weight you want. Then label each one with the correct weight.

Another way, besides using hand weights, to create resistance is to get some long strips of surgical tubing from a drug store or medical supply store, or some thick rubber bands made especially for exercising. These stretchy items act like long springs and they can be an effective substitute for expensive fitness machines.

A few accessories round out your at-home equipment: two sturdy chairs, a heavy table, a bench, a stairway step or a heavy block of wood, and a kitchen counter.

A Word about Breathing

When you are doing strength exercises of any kind, proper breathing will enhance your performance and comfort level. The procedure is quite simple: blow out during the hard part, breathe in during the easy part. Most people find that a controlled exhalation works best; that is, tighten your mouth so that the air in your lungs can be released gradually over the period of exertion (usually

203

just a few seconds). This is in contrast to keeping your mouth relaxed and allowing all the air in your lungs to be expelled instantly. The important thing is to remember to breathe while doing the exercise.

Strength Exercises You Can Do at Home

There are more than a hundred recognized strength exercises. Here are some of the best ones you can do at home:

Your Lower Body

Squat

a. Stand erect in front of your kitchen counter with feet about shoulder-width apart, toes pointing straight forward, hands gripping the counter for balance. **b.** Keep your back straight and your heels flat on the floor. **c.** Slowly bend your knees,

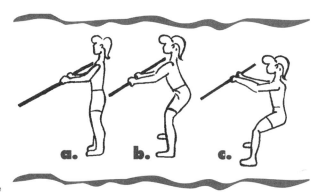

up to 90° angle if comfortable (thighs will be horizontal), while pressing down on little toes and keeping knees over feet as much as possible. Then straighten to original position. (See the detailed description of squats in Step 38.)

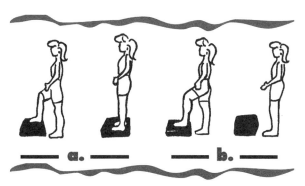

Step-Up

Find a low bench or stair about a foot high. Make sure it is stable enough to hold your body weight. If using a stair, make sure the flat part is wide enough to place your whole foot on it.

a. Start by lifting your right foot on the step; then lift your left foot onto the step also. **b.** Then come down with your right foot, then, your left. Repeat this, starting with your right foot first, for the desired number of times. Then do the same thing starting with your left foot. You can increase the resistance by increasing the height of the step or by holding hand weights at your sides.

Stationary Lunge

a. Stand with feet slightly apart, toes forward, knees relaxed and arms down at your sides. **b.** Move one foot forward with back leg balancing on ball of back foot. Your back heel should be off the floor and your back knee should be

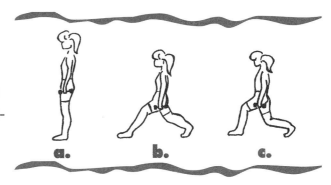

205

slightly bent. This is your starting position. **c.** Next, start lowering your body to the floor by bending your front knee. It's important to come down as if you are balancing a jug of water on your head (shoulders over hips, front knee aligned with front foot). Keep your arms at your sides. Return to the starting position **(b)** and repeat for the desired number of repetitions. Then change legs and repeat this exercise. For the advanced version, hold dumbbells at your sides.

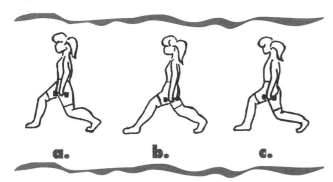

Walking Lunge

A walking lunge is like the stationary lunge above but with more motion. This variation is more advanced and really challenges your balance.

a. Start with arms down at sides and lower your body as you would for a stationary lunge (head over shoulders,

shoulders over hips, front knee aligned with front foot). **b.** As you come up, spring forward with your front leg and move your back leg to the front, **c** lowering your body as before. Indoors, it is best to do these in a long hallway so you can keep going in a straight line and focus on your form. For the advanced version of this exercise, hold dumbbells at your sides.

Calf Raise

Place your feet on a block of wood or on a step so that the toes and balls of your feet are supported but that the heels extend over the edge. Have a counter or sturdy railing to hold onto for balance. **a.** Keeping your

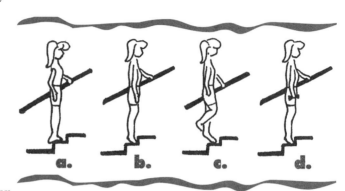

206

body straight upright, sag your heels as far below your toes as possible. **b.** Raise up on the balls of your feet as far as you can, then return to the starting position. This should be done slowly and smoothly. Make sure your ankles do not roll outward as you do this. **c.** For the advanced version, do one leg at a time by wrapping your other foot around the ankle to be raised, or **d.** use a dumbbell in the hand corresponding to the foot being worked.

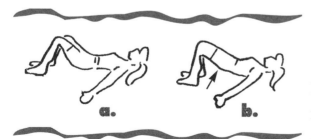

Bridge

a. Lie on your back with your arms straight out at your sides, with both knees bent and both feet flat on the floor. **b.** Keeping your upper back on the floor, slowly raise your buttocks until there is an imaginary straight line from your shoulders to your knees. Then slowly lower your pelvis back to the floor. Don't arch your back. Repeat this for the desired number of repetitions. For a variation on this exercise, place a ball between your knees and squeeze the ball as you come up and down. This works your inner thighs.

Your Back
Bent-Over Row with Dumbbells

a. Stand to the left of a flat bench or stable chair, with a weight in your left hand. Extend your left leg back about 18 inches to the rear and keep both knees bent. Bend over from the hips, place your right palm on the bench or chair seat for support and to brace

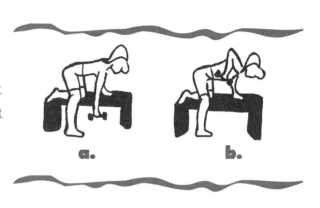

your torso, keeping your right elbow slightly bent. **b.** With your left hand held so the palm is facing your body's midline, slowly pull the weight up until it lightly touches the side of your rib cage, pulling your left shoulder blade back at the top of the movement. Slowly lower the dumbbell back down to the starting position. Do the mirror image of this, with the weight in your right hand.

Seated Row with Elastic Tubing

a. Sit on the floor with your legs out in front of you, keeping your back straight. Wrap elastic tubing around your feet and hold the ends of the

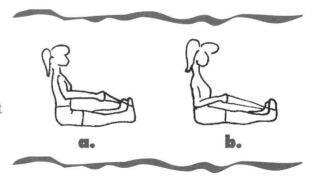

tubing in each hand, with your arms extended in front of you. **b.** With your knees slightly bent, slowly pull your arms toward your waist, pushing your chest

207

out and squeezing your shoulder blades together. Keep your abdominals tight so that your lower back doesn't arch. Slowly return to the starting position and repeat for the desired number of times. You can make this exercise harder by shortening the length of elastic tubing (wrap more of it around your hand).

Modified Pull-Up

a. Lie on your back under a heavy and sturdy table. **b.** Grasp an edge of the table firmly and raise your body, using your arms (be sure the table doesn't tip). Go as far up as possible, then sink evenly back down again. Make sure your arms come back

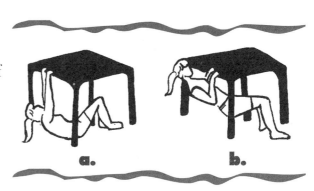

down all the way between repetitions. For the beginner level of this exercise, keep your legs bent at the knees. For the advanced level, keep your legs straight and use a wide grip (your hands gripping opposite edges of the table if possible).

Chest

Dumbbell Press

a. Grasp two dumbbells and lie on your back on a flat bench, your knees bent and your feet flat on the bench. The dumbbells are held at your sides by your chest. **b.** With your eyes looking up at the ceiling,

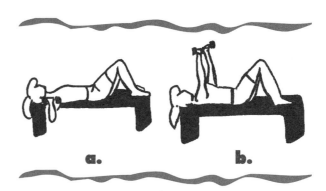

slowly raise the dumbbells over your chest (over nipple line) until they come together. Elbows should be slightly bent. Then slowly bring them down. Repeat for the desired number of repetitions.

208

Push-up

Push-ups can be done in any of three levels of resistance.

Level I: Wall Push-Up

a. Stand about an arm's length away from a wall, palms against the wall about chest height, knees slightly bent.
b. Keeping your neck, head and back straight and your abdominals tight, slowly bend your elbows and lean forward, until your forehead touches the wall. Pause for a second, then use your arm and shoulder muscles to push back to the starting position.

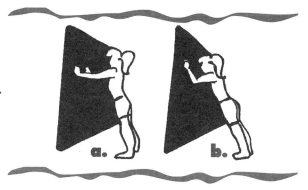

Level II: Modified Floor Push-Up

a. Kneel on all fours on a padded floor, hands about shoulder-width apart and positioned slightly forward of your shoulders, feet facing back with toes flat on the floor. Press your hips down to keep your torso in a straight line and keep your abdominals pulled in. **b.** Slowly bend your elbows and lower your body as a unit, chest and chin moving down to nearly touch the floor. Then push back up. Don't lock your elbows.

209

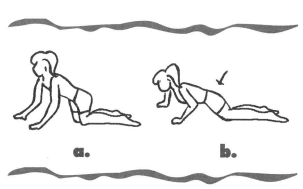

Level III: Standard Push-Up

a. On a padded floor, balance your weight on your hands and feet. Hands are about shoulder-width apart and positioned slightly forward of your shoulders.

Your legs are extended straight back, supported by the balls of your feet. Keep your torso in a straight line. **b.** Slowly and smoothly bend your elbows and lower your body as a unit, chest and chin moving down to nearly touch the floor. Then push back up. Don't lock your elbows.

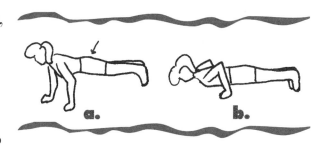

Shoulders

Prone Lateral Raise

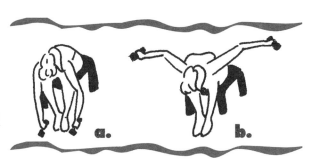

a. Sit in a chair or on a bench, your knees apart, your back straight, your feet spread about shoulder-width and flat on the floor. Your arms are at your sides, grasping light dumbbells. Slowly bend forward at the hips, and, if comfortable, try to rest your chest on your thighs. You should keep the arch in your back as you bend forward.

b. Keeping your head and chest down, start raising your arms slowly upward as if a string is pulling them up by the wrists. Keep your elbows slightly bent. Raise arms as high as comfortably possible, pinching shoulder blades together, and then bring them slowly down. Repeat this exercise for the desired number of repetitions. If it hurts your back to be bent forward, you can do the alternate lateral raise described below.

Alternate Lateral Raise

a. Lie on your side with your legs straight and your top arm stretched out in front of you. **b.** Hold a light weight with your top hand and slowly

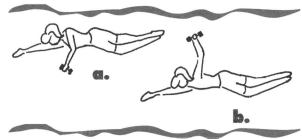

raise your straight arm toward the ceiling. Do not go beyond your body's midline. Slowly bring your arm back down. Repeat for the desired number of repetitions, then turn onto your other side and lift your other arm.

Arms

Bicep Curl with Dumbbells (for front of arm)

a. Stand or sit erect, elbows pulled into sides. Grasp the weights with your hands, palms facing forward. **b.** Keeping your elbows at your sides, bend your arms and pull the weights up to your shoulders. Then slowly return to the starting position.

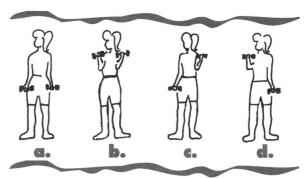

a.   b.   c.   d.

211

   You can also alternate arms for this exercise (**c** and **d**). Make sure your arms come back down all the way. Repeat for the desired number of repetitions.

Tricep Kickback with Dumbbells (for back of arm)

a. Standing next to a bench, grasp a dumbbell in your right hand. Bend forward until your left hand is on the bench, supporting your back.
b. Begin with your right arm bent at a right angle and without moving your elbow, slowly move your arm back and up until it is straight.
c. Slowly return to the starting position. As you do this, keep your arm against the side of your torso. Do the desired number of repetitions, then switch to the other arm.

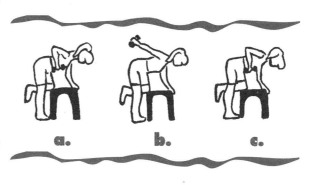

a.   b.   c.

Tricep Extension with Dumbbells

a. Standing or seated erect, grasp one weight with both hands, palms up, and bring your arms straight up overhead. Hold the dumbbell vertically, with the thumb and index fingers of each hand, with one hand below the other. **b.** Bend your elbows, lowering the weight behind your head. **c.** Then straighten your elbows, pushing the weight up overhead again. Keep your arms close to your ears throughout this exercise.

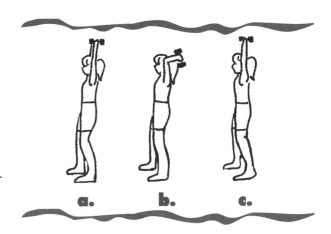

Modified Dip, with Two Chairs

a. Place two chairs about 24 inches apart, facing each other. Bend your knees and place your feet on the floor directly beneath your buttocks between the two chairs. Hands are pointed forward on chairs with elbows pointing behind you. **b.** Using your arm muscles, slowly push yourself up just far enough to almost straighten your arms but not far enough to lock your elbows. **c.** Then, using your arm and leg muscles, begin lowering yourself, elbows pointing behind you, until you feel your chest muscles beginning to stretch. As you lower yourself, keep your shoulders down—don't let them rise up to ear

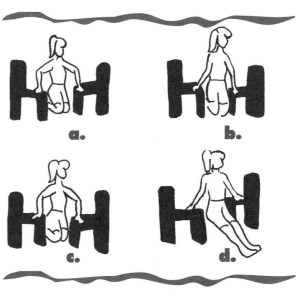

212

level. Don't lower yourself beyond the point where your shoulders are at the level of your elbows. Repeat for the desired number of repetitions.

In the beginning, use your legs to help raise and lower yourself. Over time use your legs less and less, until you can eventually extend them in front of you (advanced level—see picture **d**).

Some Things to Remember

- Incorporate strength training into your fitness program. At least 6 different exercises, 2-3 times per week.
- Do 1 or 2 sets of 12–15 repetitions.
- Your last 3 reps should be hard to do. When they get easy it's time to increase the weight.
- It's better to have your body balance and stabilize itself than to use a machine.
- Breathe! Exhale during the hard part of the exercise and inhale during the easy part.
- Rest your muscles at least 48 hours after strength exercises. If you work your muscles really hard, rest them for 72 hours.

213

STEP 42 — **Stretches**

Our typical modern daily routine of tasks and pleasures does not sufficiently stretch our bodies. Part of this is natural aging of the body—it is hard for an adult to maintain the suppleness of a young child. However, if every day we carried water from a well to the house, sought fleet-footed game and needed a high degree of nimbleness to create our artifacts, we would be able to maintain much of our early flexibility. But we no longer do those things—our modern lifestyle has made us largely sedentary.

When we don't regularly stretch our muscles and connective tissues, they tend to lose their elastic ability. The result is that, for most of us, each year we become more stiff, less flexible, with less range of body movement. In turn, this reduces circulation and makes us more brittle—more prone to disease and injury.

We need to compensate for this with a formal program of stretches, but we need to do it right. When your muscles have been at rest and are relatively cool, their ability to stretch beyond the positions they are used to is limited. If you do stretch cold muscles, it does more damage—your muscle fiber is likely to be torn. But when your muscles are warm they are looser, and the muscle fibers can bend and stretch more easily. That is why it is so important to stretch *after* you warm up or better yet, after you exercise, because your muscles are warm and loose and are ready to be stretched.

When you do stretches, always stretch slowly and gradually up to a point of tension. What is a point of tension? It's the point just beyond what is comfortable but not far enough to cause pain or hard strain. The correct tension point is where you feel your muscles pulling just a bit beyond what they're used to. Never stretch beyond the tension point to where you feel pain. When you reach

When we don't regularly stretch our muscles and connective tissues, they tend to lose their elastic ability.

214

the tension point, hold that position for 30 to 60 counts. Never bounce; that is, don't go back and forth between relaxed and stretched positions—that doesn't improve your flexibility and is more likely to cause injury. Added flexibility comes from keeping your muscles stretched—without movement—for at least a minute.

Okay, now you're ready to try them. Here is a list of stretches that will help keep you flexible and healthy. You can do each one a single time or as many times as you like.

Neck

a. Stand erect, with your arms dangling at your sides. Tilt your head to your right side. Lower your right ear toward your right shoulder while keeping your shoulders down. Hold this position. Then repeat to the left side. **b.** Turn your head to the right with chin pointing toward shoulders (shoulders remain still). Hold this position. Repeat this to the left side. **c.** Pull in your chin to make a "double" chin, stretching the back of your neck. Hold this position. **CAUTION: Do not lift your chin up and tilt your head back while doing this—it hyperextends your neck.**

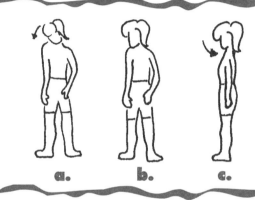

215

Shoulders

Move your shoulders in a circle.
a. Start with five forward circles,
b. then five backward circles.
c. Stretch your right arm across your chest with your left hand pressing against your right shoulder. Hold this position. Repeat with left arm.

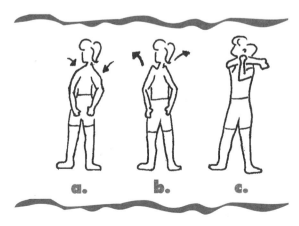

Chest, Shoulders, Neck and Posture

a. Touch the middle fingertips of both your hands behind your head. Slowly pull back your elbows, squeezing your shoulder blades together. Hold 20 to 30 seconds, then relax. **b.** Lower your chin toward your chest, gently pulling your elbows forward. Hold this an additional 20 to 30 seconds. **c.** Stand with your chest up, shoulders back, feet shoulder-width apart and knees slightly bent. Clasp your hands together behind your lower back, palms inward. Slowly and gently push your arms upward until you feel mild tightness. Do not bend at the waist or round your shoulders.

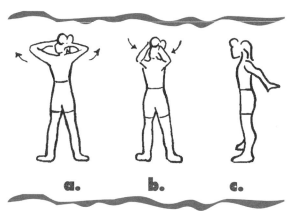

a. b. c.

216

Posture Stretch for Sitters

a. Lie on your stomach with your palms on the floor slightly forward of your shoulders. Relax your back, and slowly press up your body for a good back and abdominal stretch. Keep hips on floor and eyes looking straight ahead (not up). Hold this position. **b.** Then lower yourself. In the event of lower back pain, either do not lift as high or discontinue stretch.

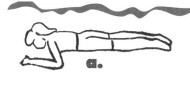

a.

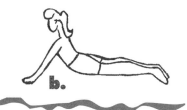

b.

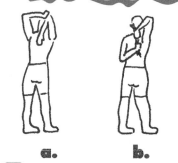

a. b.

Triceps (back of arms)

a. With your left hand, pull your right elbow behind your head. Your right elbow will be sticking straight up behind your head. With your left hand gently pushing down on your right elbow, stretch the fingers of your right hand down your back. Hold this position. Then do the same on the other side.

b. For a deeper stretch, grasp a towel with your right hand and bend your right elbow, dangling the towel down the center of your back. Place your left hand behind your back and reach up to grab the towel end. Gradually move your hands closer together. Hold this position. Then do the same on the other side, alternating your hands.

Upper Back

a. Bending your elbows, interlock your fingers in front of your chest, palms outward. **b.** Push your arms forward, straightening your arms and rounding your upper back. Hold this position.

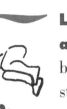

Lower Back

a. Lying on your back with your knees bent, feet flat on the floor and your arms straight out to the sides, bring your knees toward your chest and keep them bent at a right angle.

b. Keeping both shoulders on the floor, slowly let your legs fall to the right side until your right leg is resting on the floor. Hold this position. Then repeat on the other side. **c.** Get on your hands and knees. First arch your back up like a scared cat. Pull your stomach in and hold this position. **d.** Then lower your back until it bows in the middle. Hold this position. Repeat as many times as you like.

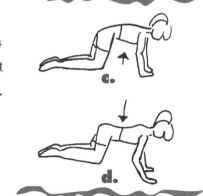

217

Hips

Lie on your back with your legs together straight in front of you, resting on the floor. **a.** Clasping your hands under your right thigh, gently pull your right knee to your chest while keeping your left leg straight in front of you. Hold this position. Then repeat with your left knee. **b.** Lying on your back with your right foot flat on the floor, place your left ankle over your right thigh. Clasping your hands under your right thigh, gently pull your right knee towards your chest, using elbow pressure to keep your left knee pressed out. Hold this position. Then repeat with your left leg.

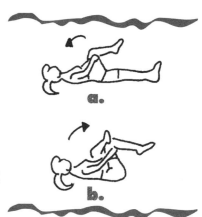

218

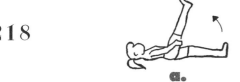

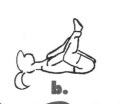

Hamstrings (back of upper leg)

a. Lying on your back, slowly raise your right leg, clasping your hands under your right thigh. Your left leg is straight with heel resting on the floor. Gently pull your right leg toward your chest, keeping it straight. Hold this position. Repeat with your left leg.

Inner Thighs

b. Lying on your back with your knees apart, grasp your ankles with both hands and gently pull your feet toward your chest. Use elbow pressure to keep your knees apart. Your upper body should be relaxed. Hold this position.

Quadriceps (front of upper leg)

a. Lie on your left side with your legs straight and your left knee bent slightly forward. Grasp your right foot or ankle with your right hand and gently pull your right knee backward without arching your back. If you are not

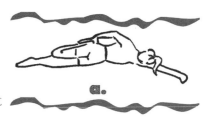

troubled by knee problems, pull your right heel gently toward your buttocks during this stretch. Hold this position. Then repeat for the other side.

Hip Flexors

a. Get down on your left knee as if you were going to propose marriage. Your right knee should be at a right angle to the floor, with the knee over the ankle. **b.** Without moving your right leg, press your hips forward until you feel a stretch in the upper part of your left thigh. Don't let your back arch. Repeat with the other leg.

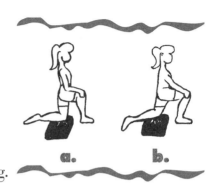

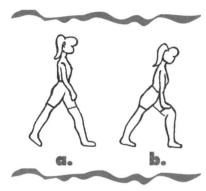

Calf

a. Stand erect, with your arms dangling at your sides. Step forward on your left foot, with your right leg resting on toes pointed straight forward. **b.** Press your right heel to the floor, keeping your left knee aligned over your left ankle. To feel more stretch, slide your right foot farther backward. Hold this position. Repeat for the other side.

219

Achilles

a. Begin with doing a calf stretch **b.** and then slightly bend your back knee without lifting your heel. Hold this position. Repeat for the other side.

Some Things to Remember

- Stretch regularly.
- Stretch when your muscles are warm and loose.
- Stretch slowly and gradually, up to a point of tension.
- Never bounce!
- Hold the stretched position for 30–60 seconds.

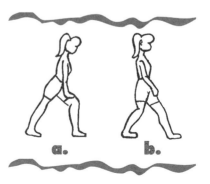

At Home or at the Fitness Center?

Strength and aerobic exercises can be done either at home or at a fitness center; each has its advantages and disadvantages. Modern fitness centers have a wide variety of equipment . . . often two or three different machines for doing essentially the same thing. Some people love the variety, the companionship and the structure of a workout at a fitness center (by structure, we mean that it's harder to procrastinate at a fitness center because there's nothing else to do). Others are embarrassed if they are watched while exercising, or just by appearing in public in a workout suit, especially if they are out of shape.

On the other hand, if you exercise at home you can do it pretty much whenever you want to, and you can do it to your own favorite music or TV show. However, you need adequate space. A room dedicated solely to exercise is ideal, of course, but few of us have that. But how much furniture moving do we have to do each time we start and stop exercising? If it is a lot of work to prepare the room for exercise, and then return it to its normal condition when we're finished, it's unlikely we'll keep it up for long.

If you prefer to exercise at home, do keep your exercise space clean and tidy. The flooring is important. If your exercise room has just a bare, hard floor, you won't look forward to lying on it—especially if it's cold in the winter. Get a small piece of rug that you can roll up when you're finished.

If you decide moving furniture around isn't for you, but you are a little shy about exercising at the fitness center, there are some things you can do to help make your workout experience more pleasant and effective. Here are some tips:

- Find a friend to go with you.
- Go to the fitness center during quieter hours (usually, late mornings and early afternoons on weekdays are best).
- Wear clothes that are comfortable. You don't have to go around in a skimpy leotard or have the latest fashion workout suit.

220

- Take a book with you to keep you company, or a miniature radio or cassette player with earphones.
- Make an appointment with a trainer at the fitness center to make up your routine.
- Make sure you are comfortable with your routine and that you can easily follow it.
- Do your aerobic exercise before strength exercises so that your muscles are warmed up.
- Find a quiet corner or other spot where you can stretch and do floor work.

There is another aspect to the question of exercising at home or at a fitness center. When you use machines to create the resistance for a strength exercise, you are usually sitting, lying down or otherwise firmly connected to the machine. When you create resistance by using your body alone, you gain the added benefit of enhanced coordination and balance—your body is controlling more of the exercise than is possible with a machine.

Having said this, the choice is still yours. Whatever helps you to stay regular with your program is the right thing for you.

Fitness Classes

Classes have several advantages. The obvious ones are that you feel more committed, more obligated to your exercise program when you are part of a formal group, and it is easier to plan time for your exercise when you have a class schedule. You will also probably meet one or more persons in the class with whom you can share mutual encouragement.

Beyond this, there is another distinct advantage to a class; the program is consistent, week after week, and you are much less prone to deviate when some minor inconvenience comes along.

Some "beginners" classes may actually be for beginners while others are

221

more advanced; same goes for all levels of classes. Before you join a fitness class, be sure to check it out first by visiting the group or, if that's not possible, talking to the instructor.

Exercising with a Buddy

For most of us, almost everything is more fun when we have someone to do it with, and it's especially true with exercise. But more than fun, your chances of staying with your exercise program are greatly enhanced with a companion. There'll be days when the last thing you want to do is exercise, but you'll do it because you don't want to disappoint your buddy. And when you both see the beneficial effects your exercise is having on each of you, you will reinforce each other's resolve to keep going.

If part of your exercise program includes walking, for example, it's usually not hard to find someone who will walk at your pace. On the other hand, if your partner needs to exercise at a level below or above you in other activities, it can prevent you from performing at your own correct level. So it's important to find someone whose ability matches yours.

If you're having a hard time finding someone to exercise with, try putting a note on the bulletin board at your local fitness center, spa or church. Give this a high priority—there is a strong chance that your success will depend on it.

The Advantages of a Personal Trainer

Why pay for the services of a personal trainer? In all skilled fields, from concert pianist to professional basketball player, everyone benefits from professional guidance. In the area of fitness, as well, a competent trainer can be very helpful. For example, exercise programs need to vary with the individual. A good trainer will know what kinds of exercises and routines will work best for the shape you are in right now, and the most effective routines that fit your schedule and goals. As you progress, different exercises and/or equipment may be needed, and your

222

trainer will recommend the appropriate changes. This can speed up the results and make your experience more pleasant.

When you are engaged in an exercise program, all sorts of questions come up: What eating habits will complement your exercise program? What's the best way to treat a strain, a sprain, a cramp or generally overworked muscles? A competent trainer will be able to answer your questions as they arise—right when you need to know—not after the fact, when some damage may have already been done.

Your trainer should know how to challenge and encourage you, to keep you motivated, without overloading you or creating unrealistic goals.

How do you find the right personal trainer? As recently as five or six years ago, the image of a fitness trainer was someone with bulging muscles who looked great in tights. Today that image has been replaced by individuals who are educated and highly skilled in exercise physiology, biomechanics, nutrition, stress reduction, exercise safety and sports medicine, to name a few related subjects.

For a start, make sure your prospective trainer is currently certified as a "personal trainer." While there are a large number of certifying organizations, here are the best-known, most reputable ones.

- American College of Sports Medicine (ACSM)
- Aerobics and Fitness Association of America (AFAA)
- National Academy of Sports Medicine (NASM)
- National Strength and Conditioning Association (NSCA)
- The Cooper Clinic
- American Council on Exercise (ACE)

At the time of this writing, personal trainer certification is unregulated by the states. While there are dozens of excellent, local certification programs, there are also many that are questionable. If your trainer has been certified by one of the above organizations, you can have confidence in his or her technical ability.

Beyond fitness knowledge, however, is whether you and your trainer work

223

well together. It's not just if you like each other or not. The right personal trainer will help coax the very best out of you, and that ability to do your best will serve you in every area of your life.

Whether your choice is a personal trainer, a fitness class, or one or more exercise buddies, do find a way to exercise with others.

One Type of Exercise Won't Do It

Walking, weightlifting and yoga—representing aerobic, strength and flexibility exercise, respectively—are all beneficial, but each by itself will not bring you to a high level of fitness. Include a variety of exercise activities in your overall routine, including at least one aerobic activity, and an appropriate mix of strength and flexibility exercises.

Making It Fun

Some of the things that make exercise fun are: good companionship; music; listening to books on tape; reading (we know of several individuals who read or watch TV while exercycling and a few who read the paper while walking on the treadmill); competitive sports; and beautiful surroundings. What makes it fun for you? If you don't yet know, find out and do it!

Let's Hear It for Music

Add music to your chores. Start by compiling some tapes, CDs or records that are so snappy and lively, you can hardly stand still when you hear them. Play them when you're cooking, doing dishes, vacuuming or taking care of other household chores, and let yourself move with the music. It will make your chores more fun and it will burn calories.

Fitting Your Exercise Routine into Your Life

If your exercise routine is too disruptive, not only will you be tempted to forego it, you'll probably begin to resent it. Take some time for careful planning. Most people have some leisure time during the day or evening during which they're used to being sedentary—watching TV, etc. Maybe you can use your leisure time for exercise; this will cause a minimum of disruption to your other obligations.

The critical thing in fitting an exercise routine into your life is what priority you give it. If you give it a low priority, so that reading the newspaper, chatting with a friend or shopping for new clothes are more important, chances are you won't stick to it. If you give it a high priority, maybe even right behind food and shelter, you'll succeed. Don't allow minor divergences to disrupt your routine. If the phone rings, tell them you'll call back (or turn the phone off while you're exercising). If a friend asks if she can stop by right then, tell her no. If you spot a dirty window, let it be until you're finished. If the cat insists on playing with you just then, insist right back that this is your private exercise time.

If possible, plan your fitness week. On your calendar, mark the days and times you will set aside for exercise. In general, try not to go more than two days without exercise.

If You're Bored, Change Something

Don't keep plugging away if you're not enjoying your exercise—find something that's more fun. Try changing when you exercise; where you exercise; the type of exercise you're doing; or who you're exercising with. If you can't stand a smelly locker room, change. If the swimming pool water is too cold, change. If there's too much annoying traffic on your jogging route, change.

Try cross-training. Pick three different aerobic activities you like and alternate them throughout the week.

More Physical Activity in Everything You Do

When you wake up, get physical while you're still in bed. Stretch your fingers and then your arms. Move your shoulders up and down. Bend your legs, then stretch them. If there's room in your bed, roll over in each direction. Get physical!

225

Later in the day, don't choose the closest parking place—walk a bit to where you're going. Get into the habit of taking the stairs instead of an escalator or elevator. If you're going out on local errands, can you take your bike instead of the car? Can you use your old hand lawnmower instead of the power mower? Can you crank your manual can opener rather than use the electric one? Stop looking for ways to eliminate physical activity from your daily life—start looking for ways to regain it.

Focus on Habits Rather than Results

It's like learning to play tennis, where learning the correct strokes and the proper form come before concern with hitting good shots. With a fitness program, learning good habits should come before concern over results. Results take time. So, in the beginning, it is very important to focus on developing good habits instead of closely monitoring your weight and appearance.

This Time Is for You

Like most of us, there are probably many demands on your time each day. Remember that your exercise period is time for you alone, free of other demands. It is an escape into your exercise sanctuary. *Treasure it!*

Forgive Your Lapses

There will be times—lots of them—when you don't exercise due to laziness or apathy; when the weather's too hot or too cold; when your exercise buddy doesn't show up; or when you just have too much else to do. From time to time we all do this. When it happens, forgive yourself and vow to begin again the next day. No guilt trips, no problems with self-esteem—just make a fresh start and do it.

Reward Yourself

Periodically—perhaps once a month—get yourself a new piece of clothing, treat yourself to a gourmet meal, or a night out as a reward for sticking to your exer-

226

cise program during that month. Buy yourself a good book. Enjoy a luxurious bubble bath. Do something nice for yourself; you deserve it! And put up a note in a prominent place that says:

I Did It This Month!

Building a Positive Image of Yourself

What would you look like if you were really fit? **You'd look great!**
How would you feel if you were really fit and remaining fit? **You'd feel great!**
What would it do for your confidence? **You'd be more confident!**
Your pride in your accomplishment? **You'd be more satisfied with yourself!**
Your health and vitality? **You'd be healthier and have more energy!**

227

Now put it all together and imagine yourself as all these things. It is not a question of if it will happen—merely a question of when. Because now you have all the knowledge and all the tools to make it happen.

Now it's *simply* a matter of attitude.

A Brief Note from Annette

Ever since I can remember I have been a competitive athlete—and I love it! But, I realize not everyone loves or even likes to exercise. So, I want to give all of you hesitant exercisers a little advice that might help you warm up to the idea of making fitness a *permanent* part of your life.

For me, making fitness fun is working out with a buddy, exploring nature and challenging myself to my outermost limits. Even though I don't expect anyone to work out as often or as intensely as I do, I believe what makes it fun for me can also make it fun for you. So, have a workout buddy, get out in nature and make goals to strive for, like participating in a local 5K walk.

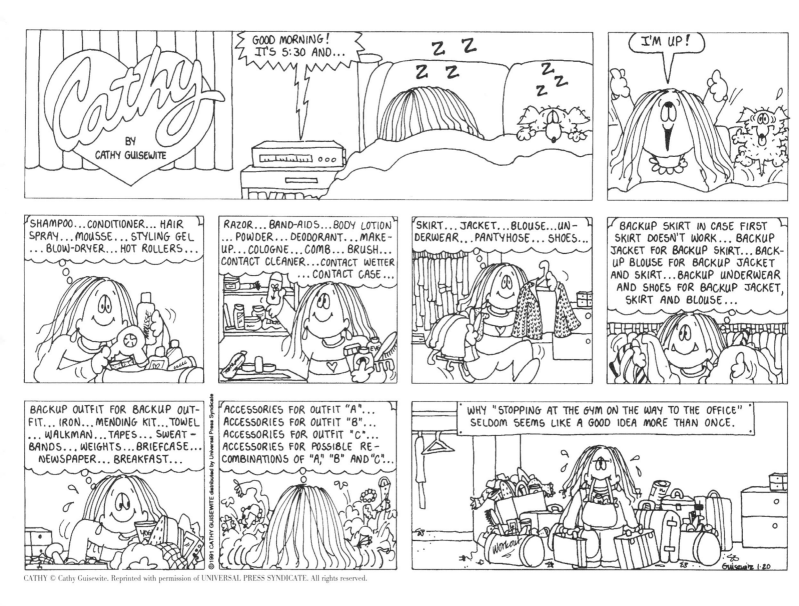

PART EIGHT

The Icing on the Cake

STEP 44 — **For Those of You Who Know What to Do but Just Don't Do It**

Changing our habits is theoretically easy. We are creatures of free will and therefore we are, or should be, free to decide how to act. And since most of us want to be healthy and trim, it is only a matter of deciding to do what's necessary in order to do it. If only it were so easy. Yet, in spite of our good intentions, we do not act in accordance with them. Why?

Are you overweight because you love the taste of food or because you subconsciously turn to food for comfort? There are many possible psychological motivations for having bad habits, but it's beyond the scope of this book to attempt to analyze them. Instead, we have focused on some practical ways to change bad habits to good ones.

In Step 27 we presented a list of food habits, temptations and triggers that have led us along the path of poor nutrition. Remember them? They included things like snacking on the wrong foods, being offered rich foods by people with whom you associate, eating buttered popcorn at the movies even though you've just had supper and feel full, and so on.

Then we suggested ways to change your eating habits. The first of these was awareness—becoming aware of your present eating habits. Next was substitution; psychologists tell us that in order to rid ourselves of bad habits we have to replace them with better ones. So we suggested good eating habits, substituting nutritious, low fat foods for fattening ones. Then we said "Practice! Practice! Practice!" because psychologists know that it takes about

66 THE REWARD OF A THING WELL DONE, IS TO HAVE IT DONE. 99

–Ralph Waldo Emerson

three weeks to really change a bad habit to a good one, and three months or more to make it automatic—so it sticks.

It's similar with exercise. In the previous steps we showed you several ways to make exercise more enjoyable and more convenient, and how to remove the discomfort associated with it. Then we told you how your fitness routine can be enhanced by exercising with a buddy, taking advantage of the knowledge of a personal trainer, and so on.

At this point, if you have read the entire book, you are equipped with all the knowledge you need to become fit and permanently reduce your weight to an ideal level. Now the question is: Will you do it and will you stick to it?

One of the elements of support is your own attitude about the success and failure of this program. When you stick to it, you gain lots of satisfaction from how good you feel and from pride in your ability. Fine. But when you don't stick to it, you must learn to forgive yourself. All is not lost when you lapse and fall back into old habits; the loss is only temporary, and you will live to win again another day. It is important to view each day as a separate challenge and opportunity; what you should be concerned with is not any one individual day, but the aggregate of days. For example, how are you doing, overall, after 30 days? 60 days? 365 days?

Another element of support is to look at what causes you, on some days, to eat improperly or to neglect exercising. Very often, the causes can be removed. For example, are there tempting foods in the house that are for other family members? If so, what can you do to lessen your temptation to eat them yourself? Be creative. Use signs and reminder notes. Buy some healthy foods that you can substitute for the less healthy ones. Make a list of alternative actions you can take when tempted.

Similarly, sometimes events conspire to make it more difficult for you to exercise. Sometimes these are of your own making. For example, you plan on working out later in the day, but then you discover you haven't packed your clothes for the gym. Can you then create one or more reminders not to make this mistake again? Remember, to affect change of any kind, the things *you do* have to change.

If it is raining hard outside and you had planned on taking a brisk walk, have you made alternate plans for indoor exercise if this should happen? If not, can you make alternate plans now so this doesn't happen again? There are usually ways to get around obstacles to exercise if we are motivated to find them.

> **You cannot change for the better if you continue doing things the same way.**

231

Often, we are very hard on ourselves and we tend to focus on our faults more than our virtues. After you begin your fitness program, keeping logs of your activities will help to put everything in a better perspective as well as help you stay in touch with your progress. Don't forget to reward yourself for doing well—you deserve it!

We all begin new programs with the best of intentions—lots of motivation and enthusiasm. Later, when we are confronted with temptations, the real challenge begins. In general, it is not the strength of your original commitment that will determine your success or failure; it is the daily system of support you have available—or the lack of it. Hey, that's important enough to say again.

The effectiveness of your daily support system will largely determine your success or failure.

Here are the elements of support:

1. Become aware of your present eating and exercise habits.
2. Remove the causes of bad habits and find creative ways to get around obstacles.
3. Substitute good habits for bad ones; use reminders to help you.
4. Don't deprive yourself of tasty, satisfying foods.
5. Make exercise enjoyable.
6. Keep logs of your eating and exercising.
7. View each day as a new and separate challenge.
8. Forgive yourself when you fail; reward yourself for progress.
9. Find a companion with whom you can share all or part of your program.
10. Practice! Practice! Practice!

232

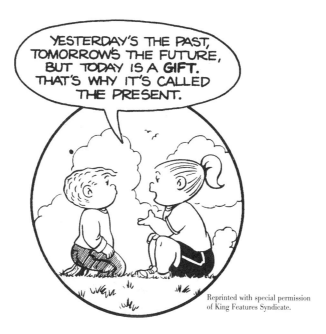

Reprinted with special permission
of King Features Syndicate.

STEP 45 — **Logs to Do It!**

In the last step, we said one of the key elements of support is keeping logs of your eating and exercising. And, since we want to be as supportive as possible, we've created a section just for logs to help you keep track. Many times throughout the book we asked you to do something like make a list, count your fats or chart your exercises. Well, this step contains a log for every little thing we suggested you do.

We hope that having these logs all together, right under your nose, will help you to get started on your program. You can even make copies of them as needed.

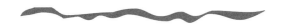

Here's a list of the logs you'll find in this step:

Fat Tracking

Pyramid Power Tracking

Plan for a Week of Dinners

Food Awareness Diary

List of Substitutions

Plan for Snack Attacks

Fast Food Options

Reward Yourself

Workout Schedule

Strength Training Log

Monthly Progress Report

Monthly Measurements

Fat Tracking

Current Fat Consumption

	ALL FAT IN GRAMS	SATURATED FAT IN GRAMS
BREAKFAST		
LUNCH		
DINNER		
SNACKS		
	TOTAL DAY'S ALL FAT IN GRAMS	TOTAL DAY'S SATURATED FAT IN GRAMS

Total Daily Fat Target: [ ]
Daily Saturated Fat Target: [ ]

	ALL FAT IN GRAMS	SATURATED FAT IN GRAMS
BREAKFAST		
LUNCH		
DINNER		
SNACKS		
	TOTAL DAY'S ALL FAT IN GRAMS	TOTAL DAY'S SATURATED FAT IN GRAMS

234

Pyramid Power Tracking for Weight Loss®

Activity Level: *Moderate*
Weight: *100–120 pounds*

The example below gives you the amounts of each food group you should eat. Just shade in each compartment of the Pyramid as you eat from the different food groups. By the end of the day, your Pyramid should be completely shaded.

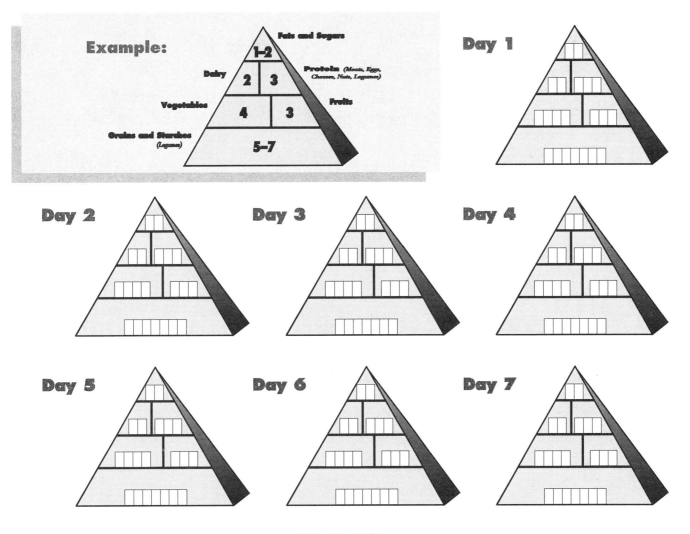

235

Pyramid Power Tracking for Weight Loss®

Activity Level: *Moderate*
Weight: *120–140 pounds*

The example below gives you the amounts of each food group you should eat. Just shade in each compartment of the Pyramid as you eat from the different food groups. By the end of the day, your Pyramid should be completely shaded.

236

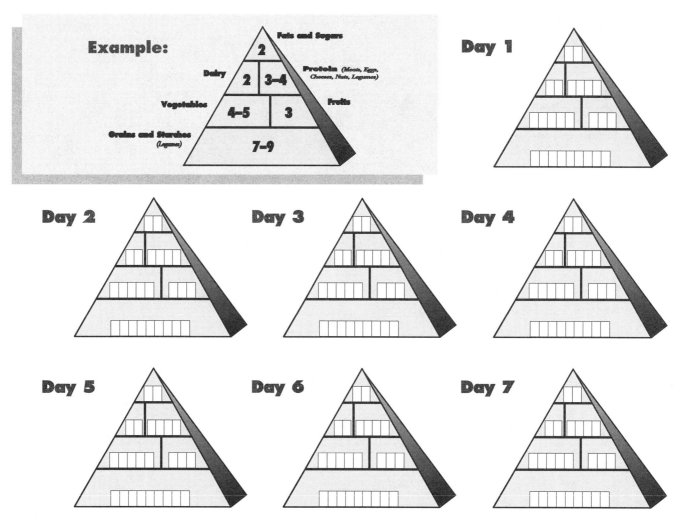

Pyramid Power Tracking for Weight Loss®

Activity Level: *Moderate*
Weight: *140–160 pounds*

The example below gives you the amounts of each food group you should eat. Just shade in each compartment of the Pyramid as you eat from the different food groups. By the end of the day, your Pyramid should be completely shaded.

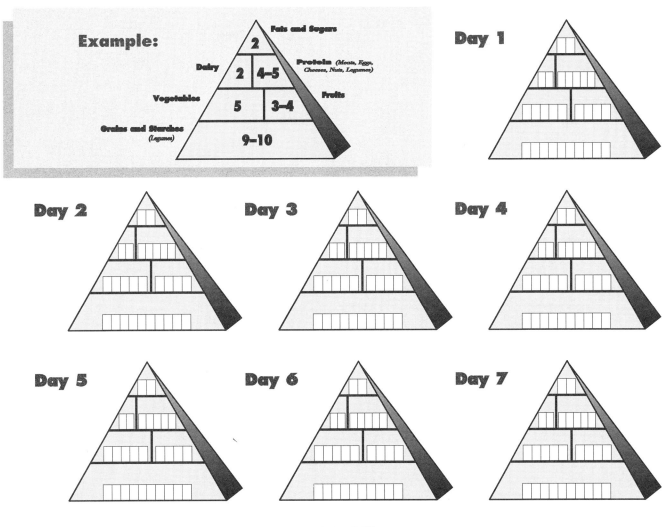

237

Pyramid Power Tracking for Weight Loss®

Activity Level: *Moderate*
Weight: *160–180 pounds*

The example below gives you the amounts of each food group you should eat. Just shade in each compartment of the Pyramid as you eat from the different food groups. By the end of the day, your Pyramid should be completely shaded.

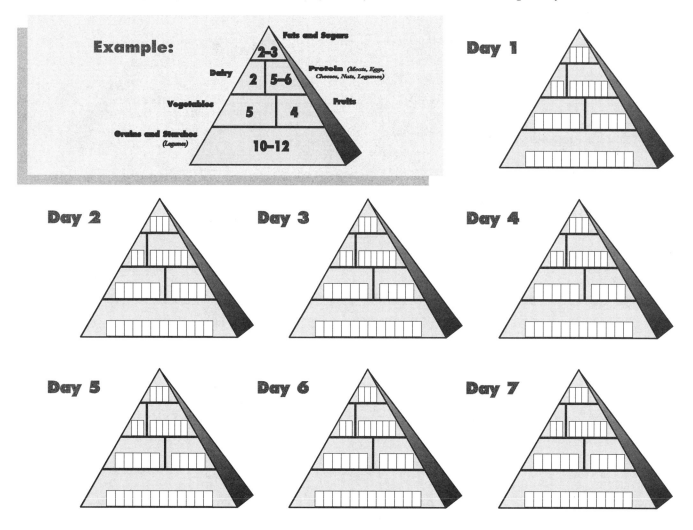

238

Pyramid Power Tracking for Weight Loss®

Activity Level: *Moderate*
Weight: *180–200 pounds*

The example below gives you the amounts of each food group you should eat. Just shade in each compartment of the Pyramid as you eat from the different food groups. By the end of the day, your Pyramid should be completely shaded.

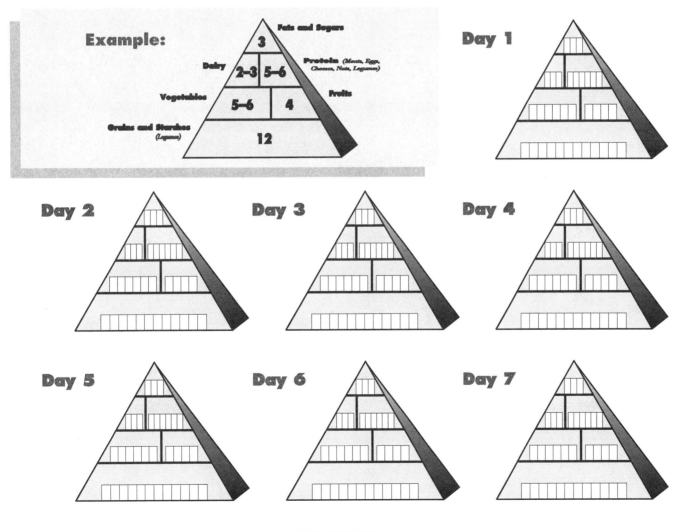

239

Plan for a Week of Dinners

DAY	RECIPE IDEA	GRAIN/STARCH	VEGGIE	PROTEIN
EXAMPLE:	Linguine & Clams with Asparagus	Pasta	Asparagus	Clams Parmesan Cheese
Monday				
Tuesday				
Wednesday				
Thursday				
Friday				
Saturday				
Sunday				

240

Food Awareness Diary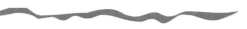

A food diary is a great tool to help you develop your sense of awareness in relation to when and why you eat. You should record everything you eat for a week to get a good idea of your eating habits and patterns.

	Food Eaten			**Situation**	
Time	**Item**	**Amount**	**Fat Grams**	**Activity**	**Feelings**
8 A.M.	bagel with jam	one/2 Tbsp.	2	breakfast	rushed

241

Remember, you want to try to eat 5–6 small meals throughout the day.

List of Substitutions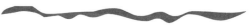

Substitution is the act of choosing and executing some desirable alternative behavior in place of an undesirable one, such as choosing nonfat frozen yogurt in place of ice cream or taking a pleasant walk instead of watching TV. You can make substitution work better if you determine, ahead of time, several substitute actions. One way to do this is to have a list of alternatives prepared for the times when you are tempted, so that right at the moment of temptation you have some satisfying options available. *Prepare this list now!*

1. _____

2. _____

3. _____

4. _____

5. _____

6. _____

7. _____

8. _____

9. _____

10. _____

11. _____

12. _____

242

Plan for Snack Attacks

This log will help you plan snacks for the three scenarios when you can have a snack attack. List your favorite healthy snacks below and then place them in your car, desk and cupboard to help reinforce your good eating habits.

243

List four snacks for your workplace drawer:

_____

_____

_____

_____

List two snacks for your car:

_____

_____

List ten snacks for your snack cupboard:
(Keep most-healthy items on lower shelves and least-healthy items on higher shelves.)

_____ _____

_____ _____

_____ _____

_____ _____

_____ _____

Fast Food Options

Make up a list of all the fast food spots along your commute drive, in your neighborhood, etc. If you have been to each of them before and you know all the items they serve—fine. If not, stop in and check them out. Each of them will probably have a few items that are low fat. For example, salads with low fat dressing, "lite" tacos, plain baked potatoes, broiled chicken sandwiches, iced tea, etc.

Then make a list of the items you can, in good conscience, get at each place. Make extra copies of your list in case you lose one. Keep a copy in your car at all times. You also might want to keep one, folded up, in your purse for when you are driving with someone else.

Promise yourself that if you do stop at a fast food place, you'll order only those items on your low fat list. Why don't you make up your list now?

244

Fast Food Restaurant: _____

Low Fat Choices: _____

_____

_____

Fast Food Restaurant: _____

Low Fat Choices: _____

_____

_____

Fast Food Restaurant: _____

Low Fat Choices: _____

_____

_____

Fast Food Restaurant: _____

Low Fat Choices: _____

_____

_____

Reward Yourself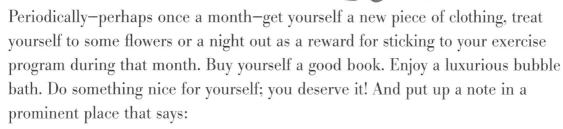

Periodically—perhaps once a month—get yourself a new piece of clothing, treat yourself to some flowers or a night out as a reward for sticking to your exercise program during that month. Buy yourself a good book. Enjoy a luxurious bubble bath. Do something nice for yourself; you deserve it! And put up a note in a prominent place that says:

I Did It This Month!

Make up a list of nonfood related rewards that make you feel special and turn to this list when you feel you deserve a treat!

1. _____
2. _____
3. _____
4. _____
5. _____
6. _____
7. _____
8. _____
9. _____
10. _____
11. _____
12. _____
13. _____
14. _____
15. _____

245

Workout Schedule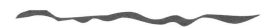

Create a workout schedule that fits into your lifestyle. Choose activities you enjoy and pick the best time of day when nothing interferes with your exercise. Be sure to have a day of complete rest, and rest between the days you strength train.

Example:

DAY OF WEEK	TIME	ACTIVITY
Monday	6:30 A.M.	Walk, 30 minutes
Tuesday	10:00 A.M.	Stationary bike, weightlifting
Wednesday		Rest

246

DAY OF WEEK	TIME	ACTIVITY

Strength Training Log

EXERCISE	DATE	SET	1	2	3	1	2	3	1	2	3	1	2	3	1	2	3	1	2	3	1	2	3	1	2	3	1	2	3	1	2	3
		Weight																														
		Reps																														
		Weight																														
		Reps																														
		Weight																														
		Reps																														
		Weight																														
		Reps																														
		Weight																														
		Reps																														
		Weight																														
		Reps																														
		Weight																														
		Reps																														
		Weight																														
		Reps																														
		Weight																														
		Reps																														
		Weight																														
		Reps																														
		Weight																														
		Reps																														
		Weight																														
		Reps																														
		Weight																														
		Reps																														
		Weight																														
		Reps																														
		Weight																														
		Reps																														

248

Monthly Progress Report

Fill in the spaces with one of the following: ■ *Needs more work*   ✚ *Doing better*   ★ *Got it down*

MONTH:	1	2	3	4	5	6	7	8	9	10	11	12	13	14	15	16	17	18	19	20	21	22	23	24	25	26	27	28	29	30	31	Total Days

EATING

aware of fats																																
watched portions																																
planned meals/snacks																																
water (8 glasses)																																
alcohol (limit)																																

EXERCISE

aerobic training																																
strength training																																
stretches																																
rest day																																

ATTITUDE

felt rested																																
motivated																																
good energy level																																

Monthly Measurements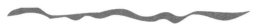

Monthly Progress

Chest measurement at start of program _____

Waist measurement at start of program _____

Hip measurement at start of program _____

Thigh measurement at start of program _____

Weight (on scale) at start of program _____

Body fat (if tested) _____

MONTHLY MEASUREMENTS					
1st	2nd	3rd	6th month	9th month	12th month

INCHES LOST!						
1st	2nd	3rd	6th month	9th month	12th month	TOTAL

STEP 46 — **Putting It All Together**

Annette: I think we've pulled it off. I think we've done it.

Joan: It's too much.

Annette: What's too much?

Joan: This book.

Annette: Come on. We've packed more information in this book than in ten other books.

Joan: That's my point. There's too much information. Look at all the other books on low fat eating and fitness—

Annette: There aren't any other comprehensive books that combine eating and fitness.

Joan: I know, I know, but how are our readers going to remember it all?

Annette: You mean like our explaining that only muscle tissue burns up body fat?

Joan: Yeah, and that's why they have to exercise regularly—to maintain their muscles.

Annette: And how their bodies try to keep them at a "set point" even if they eat less?

Joan: Yes, and why fasting actually makes it harder to lose weight.

Annette: Sure, and why "97% fat-free" isn't really 97% fat-free.

Joan: And why complex carbohydrates are so good for our readers.

250

Annette: And, of course, the Food Pyramid, and how to plan the day's and week's meals around it.

Joan: Yes, and how to read nutrition labels.

Annette: And how much fat there is in different foods?

Joan: Right, and how our readers can track their daily fat intake.

Annette: Plus, how to substitute low fat foods for high fat ones.

Joan: And learning how much each person should eat?

Annette: Yes, and how they should start using meat as a side dish.

Joan: And don't forget a really important one: how to cook with less fat without losing the flavor.

Annette: Also, the power of veggies, herbs and spices.

Joan: Can't leave out replacing bad habits with good ones.

251

Annette: Or how to eat smart when eating out, traveling or entertaining.

Joan: And something I feel strongly about—learning how to pay attention to their own needs.

Annette: And becoming more aware of their bodies.

Joan: Remember my favorite non-rule? The 80-20 Rule?

Annette: I sure do, plus showing our readers how hard they should exercise.

Joan: And protecting their backs. That's very important.

Annette: And strengthening their abs—that's important too, for much more than good looks.

Joan: And all about aerobic and strength exercises, and how to make them enjoyable.

Annette: And stretches, and developing their own exercise routines and support systems, not to mention all the great information in the appendices at the end of the book.

Joan: But that's my whole point!

Annette: What point?

Joan: It's too much!

Annette: But Joan, they don't have to remember it all. This book is to be used as a reference book . . . our readers will want to keep referring to it from time to time. Also, there's no need to remember everything—they'll be keeping logs of the most important stuff.

252

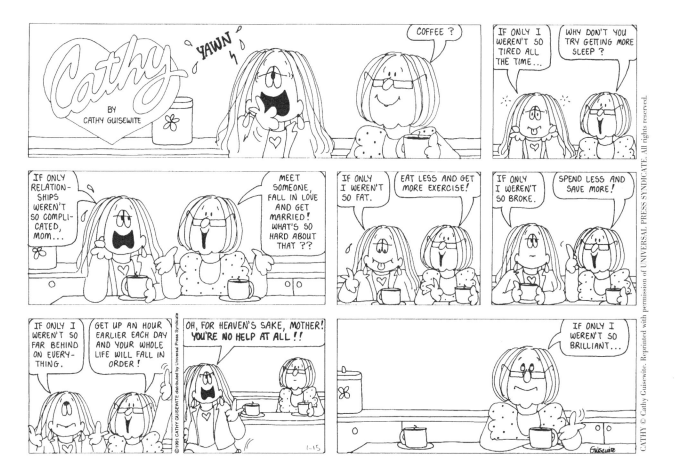

Joan: I know, I know, but I'd still like to sum it all up very simply. Maybe it would start like this: Shop low fat, cook low fat and track your daily fat intake.

Annette: That's pretty easy. What's the next one?

Joan: Plan your meals based on the Food Pyramid.

Annette: And the third?

Joan: Do moderate to hard, regular exercise.

Annette: We could call it *The Essence of Permanent Weight Loss.* Let's "note" it.

The Essence of Permanent Weight Loss

1) Shop low fat, cook low fat and track your daily fat intake.

2) Plan your meals based on the Food Pyramid.

3) Do moderate to hard, regular exercise.

253

Joan: That's pretty good.

Annette: Thanks. Now it's time for some recipes.

> ❝ A SOUND MIND IN A SOUND BODY IS A SHORT BUT FULL DESCRIPTION OF A HAPPY STATE IN THE WORLD. ❞
>
> –*John Locke*

STEP 47 — **Your Recipe for Success**

We began this book by saying that most weight-loss programs don't work. We said one of the main reasons why they don't work is that they force us to deprive ourselves of something that is utterly natural to us—good-tasting food in adequate portions. We miss it. We crave it. And sooner or later we return to the foods we want. If we've managed to lose any weight, we gain it right back—and then some. In fact, depriving ourselves of wholesome, tasty foods simply doesn't work.

But now we know what does work, and we've shown it to you in this book. We've shown you that a whole series of links have to be in place before weight loss is permanent. These are the links that have been missing from the dozens of diet plans you may have tried, and this is the reason these plans haven't worked. Here, we repeat the main ones:

- Focus on changing habits rather than on losing weight.
- Set a daily fat target.
- Learn how to prepare and eat delicious, low fat meals without depriving yourself.
- Learn how to take care of yourself.
- Understand that you can and should eat anytime you feel like it—but eat right (using the Food Pyramid).
- Know that you will lose weight permanently only as you become more fit.
- Have an ongoing fitness program that is enjoyable, convenient and effective.

This is a program that works. We have tested all parts of it extensively. If you meet your fat target, eat moderately and follow the exercise recommendations, you *will* succeed. You *will* lose weight and achieve the ideal weight for you—permanently. And your ideal weight will result in an attractive and trim body, a body that is just right for *you*. You will achieve a higher level of fitness—the actual level

254

> **"EAT NOT TO DULLNESS.
> DRINK NOT TO ELEVATION."**
>
> —*Benjamin Franklin*

will depend on how much exercise you do, from the minimum to maximum level. And your higher level of fitness will help you stay healthy and energetic. If you follow our program, you will achieve all of this without sacrifice. You'll be eating tasty, satisfying, low fat foods each day, and, based on our experience, you'll begin to look forward to your exercise routine instead of dreading it.

Fat chance of that happening? More than a chance. You can achieve the permanent weight loss you've been wanting for so many years. We know. We've done it and you can do it.

So once again, we invite you to join us. We invite you to get started—right now, on your recipe for success.

255

Joan Cortopassi and Annette Cain

A Recipe for Success
"Pitcher" Yourself Perfectly Fit!

- Mix in a tablespoon more energy burned than calories eaten, with not a single teaspoon of fasting.
- Add a generous portion of delight with inches lost but not a dash of concern for weight.
- Use complex carbohydrates without fear—they don't make you fat.
- Add a pinch of meat.
- Add a morsel of clever menu planning.
- Filter out old bad food habits and fold in new, healthy ones.
- Blend in a cup of body awareness, stretching and strengthening the muscles.
- Stir in a dollop of low fat cooking techniques.
- Add a "fresh" frame of mind.
- Pour in a cup of understanding the new food packaging labels.
- Top with Food Pyramid power.
- Drink down with eight 8-ounce glasses of water each day.
- A trace of vitamin/mineral supplements okay, but no substitute for nutritious food.
- Savor healthy living for a lifetime.

Serves: YOU!

PART NINE

Recipes (Yum!)

The recipes in this section of this book are a bit different from the recipes in traditional cook-books. While these recipes are delicious and low fat, their main purpose is to help you learn how to lower the fat in your own recipes by substituting low fat ingredients for high fat ones, and to enable you to use cooking techniques that will lower the fat in any recipe. So we recommend that you compare our recipes to those you use most often. See how you can apply our substitution methods and low fat cooking techniques to your recipes.

Now that you know how many fats you can have a day (from Step 16), you can look at our recipe nutrient information and see the fat grams per serving and decide if it fits into your daily fat target. The percentage of calories from fat has been intentionally left out. We think it makes more sense, and is much easier, to count your daily fat grams. As long as you stay within your target fat grams per day, what difference does the percentage of calories from fat make? The important thing is to count your fats.

In addition to nutritional information, each recipe also includes serving breakdowns of the different food groups. This is a tool to help you with your Pyramid tracking. In order for a food group serving to be listed, it must contain at least a fourth of a portion of that particular food.

Food servings listed are: Starch (cereal, grains, starchy vegetables and beans), Vegetable, Fruit, Protein (meats, eggs, nuts, cheese, beans), Dairy and Fat. The word sugar appears in the food serving section of recipes when two or more tablespoons of sugar are present per serving. Since we recommend you use sugar sparingly, we felt it appropriate to designate recipes with a higher sugar content.

As we outlined in Step 13, one food falls into two different food groups. That food is beans (legumes). Beans are both a starch and a protein. Whenever beans appear in a recipe, the proper food serving calculations have been made for you. We mention it again here to assist you in figuring the food servings in your own recipes.

So enjoy! And don't be shy about letting us know how you are doing. Got some good ideas for low fat cooking? We would love to see them. Send all material to:

THE COOK and THE TRAINER
11280 North Alpine Road
Stockton, California 95212

FAT CHANCE

Breakfast

Mornings are probably the busiest time of day for you. It's easy to get into the habit of grabbing something quick to eat, like a doughnut, Pop Tart, or other high fat, low nutrient food. But breakfast is an important meal. It's when you give your body its first fuel of the day. You need to recognize this and develop a strategy to make sure you get the nutrients you need to make a good start to the day.

For busy weekday mornings, pick out several smart choices that you like. For example, a whole grain bagel with nonfat cream cheese, or nonfat yogurt and fresh fruit. Whatever you decide, plan on eating a wholesome breakfast each weekday. If you plan ahead of time what you will eat, then when morning comes and you're in a hurry, you won't have to waste time deciding what's for breakfast and you won't grab an unhealthy snack item. This is something you need to give a high priority to.

On the weekends, when you have more leisure time, take advantage of it and treat yourself to a full breakfast of eggs or pancakes, or whatever tickles your fancy. Remember the 80–20 Rule: eat right 80 percent of the time and you can splurge 20 percent of the time. Of course, pancakes don't have to be splurging. They can be low in fat if you don't top them with butter. Try our low fat pancake recipe in this section and discover how delicious it can be in the morning.

On the days when you have time to prepare breakfast, keep in mind a few strategies to keep the fat low:

1. Leave the Oil Out of Pancake or Waffle Batter
Mix up a batch of batter without the oil. It really doesn't affect the flavor.

2. Control the Amount of Oil
When making pancakes or waffles, or frying or sautéing anything, spray the pan with a nonfat cooking spray or measure the amount of oil; never free-pour oil!

3. Use Substitutions
Whenever possible, substitute low fat ingredients for high fat ones. In place of eggs, use an egg substitute or a blend of egg substitute and one whole egg, or try two egg whites for every whole egg.

Monitor your fats. Know where they are.
Then relax and enjoy our breakfast recipes and experiment with your own.

258

Breakfast

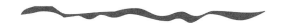

Advanced Cereal Reading

Breakfast with Bagels

Original Sunday Soufflé

Modified Sunday Soufflé

Pumpkin or Banana Muffins

Sunday Pancakes

259

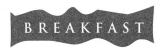

BREAKFAST

Advanced Cereal Reading

Cereal	Size	Cal	Fat
Crispix	1 cup	110	0
Raisin Squares	½ cup	90	0*
Low fat granola	⅓ cup	110	2

* Less than 1 gram

Note: If a portion has .5 grams of fat or more, the product must say 1 gram of fat, but if the portion is less than .5 grams of fat the product can claim it is fat free.

Take time to choose your cereal. If you want volume, some cereals are calculated by the ounce, some by a ½ cup and some by a cup. There is so much variety in calories and fats. You need to make the best choice for you. Do you want volume or texture?

For instance, look at the three cereals in the left column. How many fats and calories are you eating if you have 1 cup of low fat granola compared to 1 cup of Crispix? It's up to you where you want to spend your fats.

Answer:

	Size	Cal	Fat
Crispix	1 cup	110	0
Low fat granola	1 cup	330	6

260

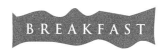

Breakfast with Bagels

4 bagels, nonfat

8 ounces yogurt, nonfat, vanilla

4 bananas

2 kiwi

Most bagels are made without egg or oil, but ask your bagel store or read the nutrition facts. If they are coated with seeds, add one fat gram per ½ slice. Any fruit can be substituted in this recipe.

Serves Eight

1— Cut one bagel in half and toast. Use a toaster oven as bagels are wide and tend to get stuck in a regular toaster.

2— Spoon 2 tablespoons of yogurt on top of the toasted bagel halves (2 tablespoons is about 1 ounce).

3— Cut a banana in half, peel, and cut into small pieces. Place banana on top of the yogurt.

4— Skin a kiwi and cut in half. Slice kiwi half and place on top of the banana.

261

Serving size:

½ bagel

Per Serving:
Calories: 113
Grams of carbohydrate: 23
Grams of protein: 3
Grams of fat: 1
1S, 1¼Fr

Original Sunday Soufflé

10 eggs

½ cup flour

1 teaspoon baking powder

½ teaspoon salt

2 cups cottage cheese

1 pound Monterey Jack or
Mozzarella cheese, shredded

¼ cup melted butter

2 cans chopped green chiles
(4 ounces each)

Serves Eight

This is the original recipe. I modified the ingredients because I didn't want to give up my Cheese Soufflé. See the compared results below. The modified recipe is on the next page. You would follow the same steps to make the original recipe as the modified recipe.

Serving size:

1 4½" x 3¼" square

Per Serving:

	Original Recipe	Modified Recipe
Calories:	518	148
Grams of carbohydrate:	9.6	13
Grams of protein:	30.6	19
Grams of fat:	**35.6**	**1.6**

¼V, ½D, 3¼P, 7Fa

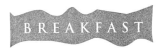
BREAKFAST

Modified Sunday Soufflé

16 ounces egg substitute

2 eggs

½ cup flour

1 teaspoon baking powder

½ teaspoon salt
(or salt substitute)

16 ounces nonfat cottage cheese

12 ounces nonfat Mozzarella
cheese

2 4-ounce cans chopped green
chiles

Topping:
8 ounces nonfat sour cream

16-ounce jar of fresh salsa

This is good to fix the day before and put in the oven the next morning. A no-fuss Christmas breakfast! Fresh fruit and lime slices look pretty with this dish and you can also serve it with a low fat sausage.

Serves Eight

1— In a large bowl, beat egg substitute and eggs until lemony in color and light in texture.

2— Add next six ingredients and stir to mix.

3— Spray a 9" x 13" pan with oil, and pour in mixture.

4— Cover and refrigerate until ready to bake.

5— Bake in a 350° oven for 45 minutes or until top is lightly browned and a knife comes out clean.

Topping:

6— Serve with a dollop of sour cream and salsa.

263

Serving size:
1 4½" x 3¼" square

Per Serving:
Calories: 148
Grams of carbohydrate: 13
Grams of protein: 19
Grams of fat: 1.6
¼V, ½D, 2¾P, ¼Fa

Pumpkin or Banana Muffins

1 cup canned pumpkin
or 2 ripe bananas, mashed

1½ cups sugar

1 cup egg substitute

½ cup applesauce

¼ cup nonfat sour cream, stirred
smooth

½ cup lite butter, melted

⅔ cup water

3 cups flour*

1½ teaspoons baking powder

1 teaspoon baking soda

1 teaspoon each cinnamon, allspice
and nutmeg

½ teaspoon ground cloves

1 cup mini chocolate chips

*Note: You can substitute 3 cups of
self-rising flour for the regular flour.
If you do this, omit the baking powder
and soda. The self-rising flour always
yields a fluffy muffin.

This is a very good low fat muffin base. You can change the flavor by using mashed bananas instead of pumpkin. To do this, use two ripe, mashed bananas and omit the allspice and ground cloves. You can substitute ⅓ cup of chopped walnuts for the chocolate chips without altering the fat content. You'll end up with a terrific, low fat banana muffin!

Serves 24

1— Preheat oven to 350°.

2— Line muffin tins with 24 paper muffin cups, set aside.

3— Mix the first seven ingredients together in a bowl, set aside.

4— In a large bowl, combine the next five ingredients. Make a well in the center of the dry ingredients and add the pumpkin mixture, stirring to combine. Add the mini chocolate chips and stir to incorporate.

5— Spoon muffin batter into prepared tins, and bake for 20 minutes, or until done.

264

Per Serving:
Calories: 154
Grams of carbohydrate: 30
Grams of protein: 2.8
Grams of fat: 2.5
1S, ¼Fr, ½Fa

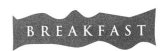
BREAKFAST

Sunday Pancakes

This is one of my favorite Sunday treats. Three pancakes, topping each layer with a little yogurt and fruit and a final topping of lite syrup. I like this breakfast for family and friends because those who want butter can choose it, and those who don't choose butter don't feel deprived.

Krusteaz Buttermilk
   Pancake Mix to make
   8 servings

1 carton nonfat raspberry yogurt

1 carton nonfat vanilla yogurt

1 banana

2 baskets raspberries

1 basket strawberries

1 basket blueberries

1 container lite maple syrup

Serves Eight

1— Put yogurts in two separate bowls for serving and place on the table.

2— Clean and prepare the fruit, then combine in two bowls for serving and place on the table.

3— Microwave syrup in two small pitchers and set them on the table.

4— Heat griddle and prepare pancakes according to directions on Krusteaz package for eight servings.

5— Serve pancakes on a large platter and let everyone decorate their own.

265

Serving size:
3 Pancakes with ½ cup fruit and 2 tablespoons each of yogurt and syrup

Per Serving:
Calories: 318
Grams of carbohydrate: 64
Grams of protein: 8
Grams of fat: 3
3S, 1Fr (sugar)

Appetizers & Snacks

Snacking is important and even healthy. It's better to eat six small meals
a day than three large ones, as this stabilizes blood sugar and gives your body
a constant fuel source throughout the day.

Keep a snack cupboard at home, a snack drawer at work and even snacks in the car.
But make sure they are healthy, low fat snacks. No nuts or potato chips—get some low fat
popcorn, nonfat pretzels, jelly beans or nonfat crackers. Then, when you're hungry for a
nibble, a good choice will be available and you won't be as tempted to go
to the vending machine or the fast food drive-through.

Try our appetizers and snacks and take them with you
to the office for a healthy, low fat treat!

266

Appetizers & Snacks

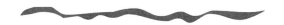

A Toast to Your Imagination
Bruschetta
Chili Cheese Torta
Dip Dip with Veggies
Fruit Dip
Hot Stuff
Nighttime Pastime
Orange Coffee Snack Mix
Tomacilantro Guacamole

267

A Toast to Your Imagination

8 ounces nonfat cream cheese

1 loaf of bread

Imaginative topping choices:

Smoked salmon or lox

Cooked baby shrimp, plain or topped with fresh salsa

Apricot or red bell pepper jelly

Leftover BBQ'd sea bass or other thick fish

Sliced mushrooms, sautéed and rendered down in white wine, balsamic vinegar, lite soy sauce and a little sugar

Roasted red bell peppers

Canned green chile peppers with low fat grated cheese

268

Your only limit with these hors d'oeuvres is your imagination. Use one or all of the suggestions in the left column.

Serves 10-20

1— Buy a loaf of interesting brown, white or sourdough bread. It can be toasted or not—your choice.

2— Trim the edges, then spread each piece with nonfat cream cheese.

3— Cut each piece into four squares or six rectangles.

4— Top with your "imagination."

5— Garnish with finely sliced green onion, other fresh green herbs, or leave plain.

6— Serve cold or hot.

Serving size:
4 squares or 6 rectangles

Per Serving:
Calories—without toppings: 79
Grams of carbohydrate: 15
Grams of protein: 2.5
Grams of fat: 1
1S

Bruschetta

1 baguette

1 ounce fresh grated Parmesan cheese

½ tablespoon olive oil

1 clove garlic, halved

3 tomatoes, Roma or pear shape, vine ripe (very ripe)

Olive oil spray

Variations:

1. If making a large batch, toast rounds using a broiler.

2. After step 5 place the tomato on first and then the cheese and broil until the cheese melts slightly.

3. After step 5 place a thin slice of Parmesan on top of baguette. Broil until slightly melted, then add your slice of tomato. Salt and pepper the cold tomato.

Serving size:
2 baguette slices

Per Serving:
Calories: 204
Grams of carbohydrates: 33
Grams of protein: 5.7
Grams of fat: 5
2S, ¾V, ½Fa

Bruschetta was the beginning of many Roman meals. It was slices of bread, grilled on charcoal, rubbed with garlic and dressed with olive oil. It was made all over Latium and Abruzzi.

Everywhere I go in Italy this is served as an appetizer and everywhere it is a little differently prepared, but the results are always wonderful.

Serves Six

1— Peel and then cut tomatoes into slices, then set aside.

2— Cut 12 half-inch-thick slices of the baguette.

3— Spray your baguette with olive oil on one side only.

4— Cut your garlic clove in half and, using the cut side, rub the clove over the baguette on the olive oil side.

5— Spray your pan with aerosol olive oil or dampen a paper towel with olive oil and coat the pan. Brown the baguettes (olive oil and garlic side down).

6— Turn them over when brown and toast the other side.

7— Place them on a plate, olive oil side up, and add a nice slice of tomato to fit on top, then sprinkle with Parmesan cheese and serve.

269

Chili Cheese Torta

16-ounce package of corn muffin mix

2 4-ounce cans diced green chiles

16-ounce can creamed corn

1 large onion, diced

2 cups low fat cheddar cheese, grated (4 fat grams per ounce)

¾ cup egg substitute

1½ cups skim milk

¼ cup vegetable oil

Vegetable oil spray

Original Chili Cheese Recipe:
Chiles, creamed corn, corn muffin mix and large onion are the same.

Changes:
2 cups cheddar cheese, grated
3 eggs, beaten
1½ cups whole milk
½ cup vegetable oil

I modified this old recipe by cutting the oil in half, using egg substitute instead of eggs, and using low fat cheese and skim milk. The result: a great old favorite with half the fat.

Serves 48

1— Preheat oven to 425°.

2— Mix all ingredients together in a large bowl.

3— Spray a 10" x 13" Pyrex dish with oil. Pour ingredients from large bowl into the Pyrex dish.

4— Bake for 50 minutes or until nicely browned on top.

5— Serve the same day or make it the day before. When serving, cut into 48 equal squares and reheat for 15 minutes in a 300° oven. It also tastes good served at room temperature.

270

Serving size:

1 square

Per Serving:

	Original Recipe	Modified Recipe
Calories:	118	87
Grams of carbohydrate:	10	10
Grams of protein:	4	4
Grams of fat:	**7**	**3**

¾S, ¼V, ½P (Modified Recipe)

FAT CHANCE

Dip Dip with Veggies

2 cups nonfat cottage cheese

2 green onions, sliced

2 tablespoons fresh parsley, snipped

¼ teaspoon dried dill or
½ teaspoon fresh dill

Salt and garlic powder to taste

Nonfat milk (as a thinner)

Suggested vegetables:

Snow Peas
Cherry Tomatoes
Jicama
Red and Yellow Bell Peppers
Broccoli

Our young grandkids like to have dip dip on their plates. It's a fun game to dip food into a sauce. It can also be a game to get kids to try food they are not sure of.

Serves 8-20

1— In a blender place cottage cheese, green onion, parsley and dill weed. Cover and blend until creamy smooth. Add salt and garlic powder to taste.

2— Chill for one hour to blend the flavors.

3— Thin with a small amount of milk.

4— Serve with your choice of vegetables.

271

Serving size:
1 cup veggies with dip

Per Serving:
Calories: 72
Grams of carbohydrate: 12.4
Grams of protein: 5.5
Grams of fat: 1
2V

Fruit Dip

1 cup nonfat raspberry yogurt

½ banana, cut into
small chunks

Assorted fruits:

Berries, whole
Strawberries, whole
Kiwis, chunks
Pineapple, chunks
Bananas, slices
Melons, chunks

Serves Six

Buy your favorite flavor of yogurt and add chunks of bananas, cantaloupe or any fruit to it.

1— Put yogurt in a small bowl, add banana chunks and stir.

2— Place bowl on a serving platter and surround with assorted fresh fruits.

Serving size: ½ cup yogurt with fruit

Per Serving:
Calories: 20   Grams of carbohydrate: 4
Grams of protein: 1   Grams of fat: Trace
½Fr

272

Hot Stuff

1 sourdough baguette

16-ounce can nonfat refried beans

4-ounce can chopped
green chiles

4 ounces low fat Monterey Jack
cheese, grated

16 ounces fresh salsa

1 bunch cilantro, washed. Pick off
30 leaves and leave the rest for
plate decoration.

Serves 10-15

1— Slice baguette into ¼" slices (approximately 30).

2— Toast on one side to make it more manageable to eat.

3— On the untoasted side, spread a layer of refried beans on all the rounds, then follow with a pinch of green chiles and a sprinkle of cheese.

4— Broil until cheese starts to melt.

5— Remove from oven and top with a small dollop of fresh salsa and garnish with a cilantro leaf.

6— Place slices on an earthenware plate garnished with cilantro.

Serving size: 3 slices

Per Serving:
Calories: 155   Grams of carbohydrate: 21
Grams of protein: 11   Grams of fat: 2
1½S, 1P

Nighttime Pastime

8 cups Crispix cereal

8 cups Corn Chex

2 cups pretzels

1 teaspoon garlic powder

2 teaspoons salt

2 tablespoons imitation
butter flakes

3 egg whites, beaten

1 tablespoon lemon juice

4 tablespoons Worcestershire sauce

Nighttime Pastime and Orange Coffee Snack Mix recipes show how egg whites can be used as an agent to coat foods with flavor without using oils. The egg white technique can be used on other recipes where you want to lower the fat.

Serves 18

1— Combine first three ingredients in a *very* large bowl.

2— Combine next three dry ingredients in a small bowl and set aside.

3— Beat egg whites until stiff, then add lemon juice and Worcestershire sauce to the egg whites. Add dry ingredients to egg whites and gently fold into mixture. Add this mixture to the cereals and toss lightly until cereal is coated.

4— Spread cereal evenly on cookie sheets and bake in a 250° oven for 1 hour. If you double this recipe it will take longer to bake in the oven.

5— Store in an airtight container.

273

Serving size:

1 cup

Per Serving:
Calories: 224
Grams of carbohydrate: 47.5
Grams of protein: 5.5
Grams of fat: 1
3S

Orange Coffee Snack Mix

½ cup sugar

1 tablespoon plus 1 teaspoon
instant coffee granules

1 tablespoon plus 1 teaspoon
unsweetened cocoa

1 teaspoon cinnamon

3 egg whites, beaten until stiff

3 tablespoons unsweetened frozen
orange juice concentrate

2 teaspoons orange rind, grated

4 cups Corn Chex or Rice Chex
cereal squares

4 cups Crispix

2 cups Raisin Squares

Vegetable oil spray

274

This is a wonderful, sweet snack, and it's addictive!

Serves Ten

1— Combine first four ingredients in a bowl and stir;
set aside.

2— Combine beaten egg whites, orange juice and
orange rind in a large bowl and stir.

3— Combine cereals in a bowl and pour into egg
mixture. Toss gently to coat, then add sugar mixture
and toss again.

4— Spray two large, shallow cookie sheets with cooking
oil spray and pour the mixture onto them, spreading
in a single layer.

5— Bake at 250° for 1 hour and 40 minutes, stirring
once or twice.

6— Store in an airtight container. Yields about 10 cups.

Serving size:

1 cup

Per Serving:
Calories: 220
Grams of carbohydrate: 49
Grams of protein: 5
Grams of fat: Trace
2¼S (sugar)

Tomacilantro Guacamole

Guacamole:

12 tomatilloes (or 1 11-ounce can of tomatilloes)

1 avocado, peeled and pitted

1 cup onion, chopped fine

2 tablespoons fresh cilantro, chopped

2 tablespoons fresh lime juice

1½ teaspoons Serrano peppers, seeded and minced

⅛ teaspoon salt

⅛ teaspoon pepper

Low fat chips:

1 package low fat flour tortillas or pitas

Aerosol oil spray

Serving size:
2 tablespoons dip with 8 chips

Per Serving:
Calories: 121
Grams of carbohydrate: 17.8
Grams of protein: 3
Grams of fat: 4
1S, ½V, ½Fa

If you prefer a smooth guacamole, use a blender after step 1. We prefer a chunky, country-style texture, so we use a masher or a fork. You can also add ¼ cup nonfat sour cream for a creamier texture without altering the fat content.

Yields 2 Cups

Guacamole:

1– Remove the paper skins from the tomatilloes and place in a dry skillet over medium heat. Heat for 3–4 minutes, shaking the pan occasionally.

2– Remove tomatilloes from heat and chop into small pieces. Place cut tomatilloes in a glass pie dish or other shallow dish.

3– Place avocado in dish with tomatilloes and mash with a fork.

4– Add onion, cilantro, lime juice, peppers and salt and pepper. Mix with a fork.

5– Use immediately or cover and chill for up to an hour.

Low fat chips:

1– Cut tortillas or pitas into eight pie-shaped wedges.

2– Spray a cookie sheet with oil and place wedges on sheet. If using pitas, spray them with oil. Bake at 375° for 5–6 minutes, or until golden. Keep the oven door open and watch chips carefully.

275

Salads & Dressings

Most salad ingredients are very low in fat; it's what we add to them that increases the fat content. As you already know, it's the dressings and some condiments like cheese, croutons and bacon bits, that contain the majority of the fat. Most dressings are fat based, from oil or mayonnaise. To lower the fat in a dressing, you must alter the base. In the Salads section of the recipes, we offer you delicious choices that are low in fat, and in the Dressings section you'll find reduced-fat, high-flavor choices to pair with your favorite salad. Here are some techniques you can use to reduce the fat in your homemade dressings:

1. Cut the Oil

Try using half the amount of oil that a recipe calls for. Adjust the tartness of the vinegar by adding a dash of sugar, fresh herbs, wine or broth. When you cut the oil in half, the resulting dressing will still have a relatively high fat content (remember there are 5 grams of fat in a teaspoon of oil), so count your fats!

2. Use the Flavor of Fruit

Fruit is naturally sweet, full of flavor and nonfat, so use this to your advantage. Try using puréed fruit mixed with fresh lemon or vinegar for a nonfat dressing alternative.

3. Substitute

As always, substitute low fat products for high fat ones. In dressings this includes mayonnaise and sour cream. Try the low and nonfat varieties of these ingredients.

4. Flavored Vinegars

Most markets now have a section of good-tasting vinegars. You can also make your own using your favorite herbs. It's a good idea to heat the vinegar before pouring it over the herbs you've selected, as this will speed up the flavoring of the vinegar. You'll find that flavored vinegars by themselves can often replace salad dressings, as they are full of flavor.

Not only salads need to be fresh—so do you! Keep a fresh frame of mind. Try our dressing recipes and the low and nonfat bottled dressings on the market, or make your own. Salads have high nutritional value and should be a frequent item in your meals—but keep them fresh, varied and low in fat.

276

Salads

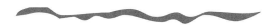

Raspberry Tomato Aspic
Summer East West Salad
Summer Pasta Salad

Dressings

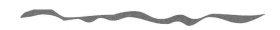

Creamy Caesar
Green Goddess Dressing
Honey Mustard Dressing
Orange Vinaigrette
Roquefort Dressing
Skinny Sandwich Spreads
Vinaigrette Dressing

Raspberry Tomato Aspic

2 6-ounce packages raspberry gelatin

2 14½-ounce cans old-fashioned stewed tomatoes

1 cup celery, diced

Dressing:

1 cup plain nonfat yogurt, strained overnight
(see Yogurt Cheese recipe on page 328)

2 tablespoons horseradish (taste and add more if you like it stronger)

278

This aspic is very tasty with almost no calories and no fat. But you won't get the taste unless you use all of the ingredients listed in this recipe. It can be a beautiful addition to a holiday buffet, molded and with dressing floated on top or on the plate.

If you don't want to strain the yogurt, blend ½ cup of nonfat cottage cheese in a food processor until smooth and add the horseradish, or use ½ cup low fat mayonnaise and ½ cup nonfat sour cream or nonfat yogurt.

Serves 15

1— Dissolve gelatin in 2 cups boiling water. **(Yes, only 2.)**

2— Cut up or blend stewed tomatoes in a blender for 1 minute.

3— Mix together celery, gelatin and tomatoes and pour into a 8" x 13" dish.

4— Refrigerate until firm.

Dressing:

5— Blend 1 cup of strained yogurt with horseradish and frost the aspic before serving.

Serving size:
1½" x 1¼" square

Per Serving:
Calories: 18
Grams of carbohydrate: 3
Grams of protein: 1.6
Grams of fat: 0
¼V

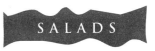
SALADS

Summer East West Salad

Marinade:

4 small green onions, chopped

1 cup cilantro, chopped

1 cup fresh lime juice (approximately 7 limes)

2 tablespoons vegetable oil

1 jalapeno pepper, halved and seeded

1 teaspoon salt

Salad:

1½ cups fresh corn kernels (approximately 2 ears)

15-ounce can black beans, drained

1 medium zucchini, diced

1 large red bell pepper, seeded and diced

¾ cup red onion, diced

1¼ pounds large shrimp, peeled, deveined

Dress plate with:

Red leaf lettuce leaves
Cilantro sprigs
Lime wedges

Serving size:

1 cup salad

Per Serving:

Calories: 246
Grams of carbohydrate: 23
Grams of protein: 25
Grams of fat: 6
1S, 2V, 3P, 1Fa

You can use this salad minus the shrimp as a cold side dish to accompany barbecued salmon in the summer— it's delicious.

Serves Six

Marinade:

1— Place all marinade ingredients in a blender and blend until dressing is smooth. The marinade can be prepared a day ahead, then covered and refrigerated.

Salad:

2— Place corn, black beans, zucchini, bell pepper, and red onion in a large glass bowl.

3— Cook shrimp in boiling water until it turns orange. Drain and reserve six large shrimp for garnish. Cut remaining shrimp crosswise into ½-inch-thick rounds, and add to the vegetables.

4— Toss with enough marinade to season to your taste and cover and refrigerate from 1 to 6 hours.

5— Before serving, arrange lettuce leaves and salad on plates and garnish with cilantro, a lime wedge and a large shrimp.

279

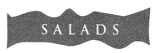

Summer Pasta Salad

Dressing:

1 cup nonfat yogurt to make ½ cup yogurt cheese *(see Yogurt Cheese recipe on page 328)*

6 tablespoons balsamic vinegar

4 tablespoons chicken stock, defatted or nonfat, or vegetable stock

1 teaspoon Dijon-style mustard

2 tablespoons fresh dill or 2 teaspoons dried dill

Salad:

1 pound penne pasta

1 tablespoon olive oil

½ medium red onion, finely chopped

2 stalks celery, peeled and chopped fine

3 ears corn, cooked and kernels removed

1 red bell pepper, roasted, peeled, seeded and chopped

6 radishes, cleaned and sliced

280

This dish can be served on individual lettuce leaves or as a large buffet salad.

Serves 12

Dressing:

1— Place all dressing ingredients in a blender and blend until smooth.

Salad:

2— Cook penne in a large pot of salted boiling water until al dente (chewy). Drain, place in a serving bowl and toss with the tablespoon of olive oil. Cool to room temperature.

3— Place the rest of the vegetables with the pasta and pour dressing over to season to your taste and toss to combine. Serve at room temperature or chill and serve later.

Serving size:

1 cup

Per Serving:
Calories: 150
Grams of carbohydrate: 26
Grams of protein: 5
Grams of fat: 2.8
1¾S, 1V, ¼Fa

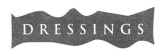

DRESSINGS

Creamy Caesar Dressing

1–2 cloves of garlic*

2 anchovy filets

1 tablespoon olive oil

2 tablespoons fresh lemon juice

2 tablespoons white wine vinegar

½ cup nonfat buttermilk

¼ cup egg substitute or 2 egg whites

½ cup nonfat ricotta cheese or nonfat cottage cheese

¼ cup plain nonfat yogurt

3 tablespoons fresh Parmesan cheese, grated

Salt and pepper to taste

*Start with 1 clove of garlic and add more to taste

Serve this dressing over cold, crisp romaine leaves, or use as a dressing for a cold pasta salad with celery, parsley and roasted bell peppers, chopped medium-fine.

Yield: 1 ⅔ cups

1— Place first nine ingredients in a food processor and purée.

2— Check for garlic flavor and add another clove if necessary.

3— Add Parmesan cheese and salt and pepper to taste; purée. Dressing is ready to serve, or can be refrigerated until ready to serve.

281

Serving size:

3 tablespoons

Per Serving:

Calories: 56

Grams of carbohydrate: 2

Grams of protein: 2

Grams of fat: 4

1Fa

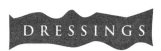
DRESSINGS

Green Goddess Dressing

1 medium shallot, cleaned

½ clove garlic

1 tablespoon parsley

1 teaspoon fresh basil

1 green onion, chopped

¼ teaspoon Dijon mustard

½ cup nonfat cottage cheese, at
   room temperature

⅓ cup low fat buttermilk

⅓ cup vanilla nonfat yogurt

1 tablespoon lemon juice

Dash of salt

Variety of lettuces

Prepare two dressings to have in the refrigerator every week. If it's ready, you will make good choices.

Yield: 1½ cups

1— Place shallot, garlic, parsley, basil and green onion in blender and chop until fine.

2— Place the rest of the ingredients in the blender and purée until you get a smooth green color.

3— Serve over your favorite combination of lettuces.

282

Serving size:
3 tablespoons dressing

Per Serving:
Calories: 32
Grams of carbohydrate: 4.5
Grams of protein: 3
Grams of fat: 0.2
No measurable food servings

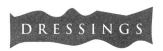
DRESSINGS

Honey Mustard Dressing

6 tablespoons prepared honey mustard

½ cup nonfat yogurt, vanilla or plain

½ cup low fat buttermilk

Honey mustard is usually a lower-fat dressing at most restaurants. Ask them how it is made.

Yield: 1½ cups

1— Place all ingredients in a blender and blend for 20 seconds.

2— Pour into a bowl or closed jar and refrigerate for 1 hour.

Serving size: 2 tablespoons

Per Serving:
Calories: 20   Grams of carbohydrate: 3.2
Grams of protein: 1.4   Grams of fat: Trace
No measurable food servings

283

Orange Vinaigrette

½ cup pulpy, "homestyle" orange juice, frozen or fresh

1 tablespoon Dijon-style mustard

2 tablespoons balsamic vinegar

1 clove garlic, cleaned and chopped fine

Salt and pepper to taste

When using this recipe, it is a nice touch to add a few orange sections or mandarin orange segments to the salad. Pomegranate seeds add a nice color contrast during the winter season.

Yield: ½ cup

1— Place all of the ingredients in a blender and blend for 30 seconds.

2— Use immediately or place in a container and refrigerate until ready to use.

Serving size: 2 tablespoons

Per Serving:
Calories: 10   Grams of carbohydrate: 2.5
Grams of protein: 0   Grams of fat: 0
¼Fr

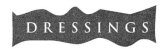

Roquefort Dressing

1 medium shallot, cleaned

½ clove garlic

½ cup nonfat cottage cheese,
    at room temperature

½ cup low fat buttermilk

⅓ cup vanilla nonfat yogurt

1 tablespoon lemon juice

1 ounce blue cheese or
    Roquefort cheese

Salt

Yield: 1½ cups

1– Place shallot and garlic in blender and chop.

2– Place next four ingredients in blender and blend until smooth.

3– Add cheese and blend until cheese is partially blended with some chunks remaining.

Serving size: 3 tablespoons

Per Serving:
Calories: 26   Grams of carbohydrate: 2
Grams of protein: 2   Grams of fat: 1
No measurable food servings

284

Skinny Sandwich Spreads

SSS #1:

1 cup nonfat mayonnaise
    (We prefer Best Foods brand)

2 tablespoons Dijon-style
    mustard

1–2 teaspoons horseradish
    (to taste)

SSS #2:

½ cup nonfat mayonnaise

½ cup nonfat sour cream

SSS #3:

1 cup nonfat mayonnaise

½ teaspoon fresh dill

2 teaspoons red onion, grated or
    1 green onion, sliced thin

Here are three different dressings to spice up your sandwiches. Adding a flavor to mayonnaise gives it some punch. You can also use these spreads as a sauce for asparagus or artichokes.

Yield: 1 cup

Instructions are for all three recipes.

1– Combine all ingredients in a small bowl and refrigerate for 1 hour to blend the flavors.

Serving size: 2 tablespoons

Per Serving:
Calories: 20   Grams of carbohydrate: 5
Grams of protein: 0   Grams of fat: Trace
No measurable food servings

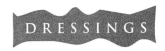
DRESSINGS

Vinaigrette Dressing

1 clove garlic, peeled

2 tablespoons olive oil

¼ cup wine vinegar, white or red

2 tablespoons hot water or chicken broth

2 tablespoons lemon juice

Salt and freshly ground pepper to taste

A normal tablespoon of vinaigrette dressing has 7–10 grams of fat. Ours has only 2.5 grams of fat.

Serves 12

1– Put the garlic clove into the blender and chop until fine.

2– Put the rest of the ingredients into the blender and blend for 20 seconds.

3– Use immediately or refrigerate until needed.

285

Serving size:

1 tablespoon

Per Serving:
Calories: 26
Grams of carbohydrate: 0
Grams of protein: 0
Grams of fat: 2.5
½Fa

Soups

Nothing tastes better on a cold winter day than a hearty bowl of soup.
And soups can be much more versatile than a winter mainstay. Summer vegetables make a
terrific base for soups, and cold soups can add pleasant variety to a warm summer day's fare.
Because most soups contain an array of fresh vegetables, they are a good choice all year long.
Here are some techniques to lower the fat in your soup recipes:

1. Replace the Cream

Cream-based soups are traditionally very high in fat. However, you can now
find some reduced fat varieties on the market. When making your own, try substituting
the cream a recipe calls for with nonfat vanilla ice cream (yes, you read it right), skim
evaporated milk, powdered nonfat milk or low fat buttermilk. And for a wonderful
taste that adds some tartness and richness to the flavor, try adding nonfat yogurt
or our Yogurt Cheese recipe to the soup base.

2. Thickness without Fat

To thicken a soup without adding fat, try removing half of the soup and puréeing
it in a blender, then adding it back to the remaining soup. As an alternative, mix two tablespoons of flour with one cup of nonfat milk and add this mixture to the soup. A third alternative
is to add a few potato flakes to soups or chilis to thicken them. A little will work wonders!

3. Final Ingredients for Flavor

In place of fatty ingredients, use flavorful herbs when finishing a soup.
These not only enhance the flavor, they add a wonderful aroma to the soup.
If you still feel the soup needs butter or oil for flavor, add only a small amount.
Limit these final additions to the minimum amount necessary.

286

Soups

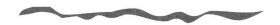

Flavorful Fungi Soup

Miso Semplice

Teresa's Minestrone

Tuscan Cannellini Bean Soup

Flavorful Fungi Soup

½ ounce dried Porcini mushrooms

1 pound fresh white mushrooms, cleaned and sliced thin

1 pound Shiitake or other style mushroom, cleaned and sliced thin

2 tablespoons butter

2 cups yellow onions, cleaned and finely chopped

2 cups Madeira

4 cups chicken broth, defatted or nonfat or vegetable stock

Salt to taste

288

This can be a rich, elegant or a rustic, country soup. At step six you can put it all in the blender if you want it completely smooth. In leftovers use it warmed over rice or use it as part of your liquid to make rice or bulgur. It can also be frozen successfully in small amounts, then used to enrich a gravy or sauce.

Serves 12

1— Soak the Porcini mushrooms in 1 cup of hot water.

2— Clean and slice 2 pounds of fresh mushrooms and set aside.

3— In a large stockpot, sauté yellow onions in 1 tablespoon of butter. When the onions are translucent and slightly browned, add 1 more tablespoon of butter and fresh sliced mushrooms and sauté for another 5–10 minutes.

4— Carefully remove Porcini mushrooms from their water and chop them into large coarse pieces. Strain mushroom water through a cheesecloth and add this 1 cup of juice to the stockpot, along with the cut Porcini mushrooms.

Serving size:

1 cup

Per Serving:
Calories: 48
Grams of carbohydrate: 5
Grams of protein: 2.3
Grams of fat: 2.5
½V, 1Fa

5— Add Madeira and broth and cook everything together for 5 minutes on high to incorporate the flavors.

6— Take half the soup out and blend in a food processor until smooth. Add it back to the stockpot. Serve in low, flat, warmed bowls.

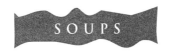

SOUPS

Miso Semplice

3 14½-ounce cans chicken broth, defatted or nonfat, or vegetable stock

2 slices fresh ginger

1 tablespoon Miso paste, red or white

¼ cup Japanese mirin (wine)

1 green onion, thinly sliced

4 whole mushrooms, cleaned and sliced

Other ingredients to add for a hearty lunch soup or a complete meal-in-one dinner soup:

Spinach leaves

Cabbage leaves, cut in narrow strips

Frozen peas

Tofu

Japanese noodles

Bean sprouts

Strips of pork cooked in the soup for 1 hour

Miso is a Japanese soy paste that can be found in better grocery stores and Japanese markets. Red Miso paste is saltier than white Miso paste. My favorite Miso is with 3 or 4 vegetables and lots of noodles, and it is a meal in itself.

If this soup is used as a starter, it's best without the noodles. As a meal, add Japanese noodles about 10 minutes prior to serving.

Serves Six

1— Open the cans of broth and using a spoon, skim off all the fat on top of the broth (if you are using nonfat broth to begin with, you don't need to do this). Pour broth into a stockpot, add the ginger slices, and cook for 15 minutes over medium heat.

2— Remove the ginger slices and add the next two ingredients. Cook for 5 minutes.

3— Slice the green onion into thin rounds. Break the stems off the mushrooms and throw them away. Cut the mushroom heads into thin slices. Place the onions and mushrooms in a small bowl and set aside.

4— Just before serving, bring soup to a boil and add the green onions and mushrooms. Ladle equal amounts into six soup bowls.

289

Serving size:

1 cup

Per Serving:
Calories: 50
Grams of carbohydrate: 4.5
Grams of protein: 7.5
Grams of fat: Trace
1P

Teresa's Minestrone

2 cups dried cranberry beans, washed and soaked for 6 hours

2 cups dried fava beans, washed and soaked for 6 hours

½ pound salt pork or bacon

1 onion, cleaned and chopped fine

5 garlic cloves, cleaned and chopped fine

4 cups water

8 quarts water (32 cups)

4 light green zucchinis, cut into 1" cubes

½ pound green beans, cut into 1" pieces

1 head celery, use heart and tender leaves only, chopped fine

4 cups cabbage, chopped

2 cups carrots, sliced

5 cups russet potatoes, ½" cubes

3 cups eggplant, ½" cubes

1 leak, heart only, cleaned and chopped

4 green onions, chopped

2 cups whole tomatoes, skinned and chopped

2 cups mashed potatoes, salted to taste

4 tablespoons pesto, homemade (*see Pestolino recipe on page 324*) or purchased (purchased pesto will increase the fat content)

Rice or pasta

Parmesan cheese

290

This is the best minestrone soup I've ever tasted. Since Teresa has no recipes, you have to stand next to her while she is cooking and write down what she does. It contains a lot of ingredients that are found in the summer, so it is a good idea to make the soup in August and freeze it in quarts or half gallons for the winter. The family can help chop and line up all the ingredients. When you thaw it and bring it to a boil, you can add your favorite pasta, broken in pieces, or a little rice.

Yield: 8 quarts

1— Soak cranberry and fava beans separately in 8 cups of water for at least 6 hours or overnight.

2— Grind up the salt pork or chop very fine and place it in a frying pan over medium-high to high heat to brown it.

3— While salt pork is browning, add onion and garlic to the pan and stir frequently on high to get everything very brown.

4— Add 2 cups of water to the mixture and bring it to a boil for 15 minutes. Pour out the water into your soup pot, reserving the pork, onion and garlic mixture and repeat one more time with 2 more cups of water. Press all the juice from the mixture so that all the flavor is in the 4 cups of water. Toss out the salt pork, onion and garlic mixture.

5– Put 8 quarts of water in the soup pot with the 4 cups of water flavored with the salt pork, onion and garlic mixture. Add the soaked, drained cranberry and fava beans to the pot.

6– Add all the chopped vegetables and potatoes and cook for 2 to 3 hours. Taste for salt. Then add pesto to the soup pot.

7– Now you can freeze the soup or use it. If you are going to use it, add fresh or dried pasta to the amount of soup you will eat and cook until noodles are done.

8– If you freeze it, freeze in the quantities that will be good for your size family; quarts or half gallons. When you are ready to use it, thaw soup and bring to a boil. Add some dried pasta and cook until done.

9– Sprinkle a little Parmesan cheese on top when serving.

291

Serving size:

1 cup

Per Serving:
Calories: 136
Grams of carbohydrate: 20
Grams of protein: 8
Grams of fat: 2.7
1S, 1V, 1P

Tuscan Cannellini Bean Soup

2 cups dried cannellini beans

Water

4 sprigs each of fresh sage, thyme and parsley

2 large yellow onions, cleaned and quartered

6 garlic cloves, cleaned

1 large carrot, cut into 4 pieces

1 celery rib, cut into 4 pieces

1 16-ounce can whole Roma tomatoes, cut in 2 or 3 pieces, plus juice of the tomatoes

½ cup white wine

3 cups canned chicken broth, defatted or 3 cups nonfat chicken broth

2 tablespoons Parmesan cheese

Salt and pepper to taste

292

This is a rustic flavorful soup that reminds me of Lucca, Italy. If you are in a hurry, you can use canned cannellini beans.

Serves Six

1— Cover beans with cold water and soak for 12 hours. Drain and rinse beans.

2— Place beans in a large pot and cover with cold water. *Do not salt.* These beans will be tender faster without salt. Bring to a boil then reduce heat to low. Cover and simmer until tender; approximately 2 hours, adding water if necessary to keep the beans just covered.

3— Strip leaves from sage, thyme and parsley.

4— Place herb leaves, onions, garlic, carrots and celery in a food processor and pulse 20 times—a medium chop. Process in two batches for a more even chop.

5— Spray a large sauté pan with olive oil. Heat pan and pour chopped vegetables into the hot pan. Sauté until brown and golden. You can spray 2 to 3 times for good color.

6— Add the cut Roma tomatoes with their juice and ½ cup of wine to the sauté pan with the vegetables.

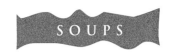
SOUPS

7– Transfer the vegetable mixture into the pot with the beans and add the broth. Stir to combine.

8– Cook over medium heat for 15 minutes to incorporate the ingredients and burn off the alcohol in the wine.

9– Take half of the soup out and purée in food processor, then add it back to the soup.

10– Cook soup on medium heat for 20–30 minutes to blend flavors and thicken the soup by evaporating the liquid.

11– Season with salt and pepper and add Parmesan cheese before serving.

293

Serving size:
2 cups

Per Serving:
Calories: 188
Grams of carbohydrate: 26
Grams of protein: 16
Grams of fat: 2
1½S, 1V, 2P

Lunch

With the rapid pace of most of our days, it's easy and convenient to eat fast food
or high fat, prepackaged items for lunch. We suggest you develop a strategy for lunch
similar to what we outlined for breakfast.

Plan ahead! Plan how many grams of fat you can have for lunch so that you meet
your daily fat target. It's really fun and challenging to have a budget and make it work.
It's just like a family budget, sometimes you're on target and sometimes you are a little off.

If you're at home for lunch, we have some great suggestions in our recipes that
are simple and delicious. Be sure you try the three dressings for sandwiches, found in the
Dressings section. They are great low fat alternatives to mayonnaise, and used this way,
they will save you 5 to 15 grams of fat a day.

There are some wonderful products on the market that are low in fat and can be heated
in a microwave when you are at the office. If you go out to lunch, we are confident that you
can find low fat choices on the menu, even at fast food restaurants. Some restaurants are
highlighting low fat choices for the customer's convenience, so they should be easy to find.
Fortunately, many restaurants are now catering to the health-conscious customer.

294

Lunch

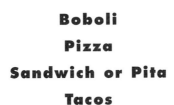

Boboli

Pizza

Sandwich or Pita

Tacos

295

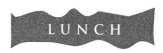

Boboli

10 fresh basil leaves or
½ teaspoon, dried

¾ cup ground whole tomatoes,
canned or fresh

16 ounce Boboli pizza crust

1½ ounces low fat mozzarella
cheese (2 grams of fat per
ounce), grated

Additional ideas for toppings:

Fresh tomatoes

Goat cheese

Green onion

Roasted red peppers

Artichoke hearts (in water)

Chopped Bruno peppers

If you add olives, use the sliced variety for better coverage and less fat. One and one-third tablespoons of olives have 2.5 fat grams.

Serves Eight

1– Chop fresh basil and mix with tomatoes.

2– Spread sauce evenly on Boboli crust.

3– Sprinkle grated cheese evenly over the top.

4– Bake at 450° for 8–10 minutes.

5– Cut into eight equal pieces.

Serving size:

1 piece

Per Serving:
Calories: 170
Grams of carbohydrate: 24
Grams of protein: 6
Grams of fat: 2.25
2S, ¼V, 1/4P

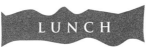
LUNCH

Pizza

1 package active dry yeast

1 teaspoon honey

¾ cup lukewarm water

2 cups bread flour

1 tablespoon milk

1 teaspoon olive oil

½ teaspoon salt

Olive oil spray

Suggested toppings:
Sautéed bell peppers

Sautéed onions and garlic

Tomato sauce

Artichokes (in water)

Sautéed mushrooms

Basil leaves

Low fat cheese, grated

Shrimp

3 fresh tomatoes, peeled and
      sautéed

Barbecued vegetables

Hot peppers

Salmon

Red onion

Nonfat cream cheese

Serving size: ⅛ pizza

Per Serving:
(Toppings are not in nutrition analysis.)
Calories: 130
Grams of carbohydrate: 2.7
Grams of protein: 3.5
Grams of fat: 1
1¾S

If you want to fix pizza for friends but want the mess out of the way, freeze the double raised dough. Allow 2 hours to thaw and proceed with your topping. It can be frozen for 3 months.

Serves Eight

1— Mix together yeast, honey, ¼ cup warm water and ¼ cup flour. Let rise for 20 minutes.

2— Add remaining water, flour, milk, salt and olive oil to the bowl of the food processor, along with your raised yeast mixture. Process for about 1 minute, until dough ball forms.

3— Place dough in bowl sprayed with oil and place in a warm spot covered with a towel.

4— Let dough rise until doubled in bulk (45 minutes to 1 hour). Punch down and let rise for another 45 minutes. Preheat oven to 450° during the end of the second rising.

5— Roll out on a lightly floured board to fit a 12-inch pizza pan.

6— Top with your favorite ingredients and bake for 8 to 10 minutes or until brown.

297

Sandwich or Pita

2 slices brown bread or 1 pita

1 cucumber

1 tomato

1¼ ounce low fat turkey
   or chicken breast without
   skin, thinly sliced

1 dill pickle

1 carrot, cut in thin slices

¼ yellow or red bell pepper, sliced

Instead of mayonnaise choose:
Mustard

Honey Mustard

Nonfat or low fat mayonnaise

Nonfat cream cheese

Skinny Sandwich Spreads
   (see recipe on page 284)

298

*If you've never tried pita bread you're missing out!
It makes a great hot or cold sandwich and is wonderful
as a chip, too. (See Tomacilantro Guacamole recipe on
page 275.)*

Serves One

1– Put your choice of dressing on 2 slices of bread,
or on the inside of the pita that has been cut in
half. Then you know how to make a sandwich–
clean, cut, slice and pile until Dagwood would be
proud of you!

Serving size:

1 sandwich or pita

Per Serving:
(Nutrition analysis does not include dressing.)
Calories: 219
Grams of carbohydrate: 35
Grams of protein: 13
Grams of fat: 3
2S, 1V, 1P

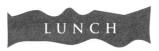
LUNCH

Tacos

1 corn or flour tortilla—
   1 gram of fat per tortilla

½ cup nonfat refried beans

½ ounce low fat cheese,
   grated

1 tablespoon canned, diced
   green chiles

 Vegetable oil spray

Other variations:
Nonfat sour cream

Chopped fresh tomatoes

Chopped green onions

Chopped lettuce

Roasted red bell peppers—
   (Mazzetta's brand have no oil)

Leftovers

A tortilla is like a piece of bread folded. You can put any-thing you want in the center. I usually use only two of the filling ingredients when I'm in a hurry.

Serves One

1— Lightly spray a large frying pan with oil.
A 2½-second spray is only a trace of fat,
or less than 1 gram.

2— When the pan is hot, lightly toast the tortilla
on both sides.

3— Take the tortilla out of the pan and place it
on a plate.

4— Place the beans on half the tortilla, then add the
chiles, then the cheese.

5— Microwave the tortilla on the plate for 1 minute.

299

Serving size:
1 tortilla with fillings

Per Serving:
Calories: 231
Grams of carbohydrate: 35
Grams of protein: 16.5
Grams of fat: 2.5
2S, 1½P

Vegetables

In the United States we are fortunate to have a large array of fresh vegetables available to us year-round in our grocery stores, farmer's markets and roadside stands. The variety makes it easy to plan healthy, low fat meals that are interesting and tasty. It's important for us to take advantage of this bounty, especially considering all the fiber, vitamins and minerals fresh vegetables contain.

In general, vegetables have gotten a bad rap. Many people think they have to be smothered in fat to taste good. This is at least partly due to the fact that many people don't know how to prepare them correctly. In Step 25, we gave several methods of preparing vegetables without a lot of added fat. You may want to review that step for menu planning with your two vegetarian meals a week.

Remember, to retain the vitamins and minerals, the texture and the flavor of fresh vegetables, light cooking is the key. Vegetables should be tender but slightly crisp after cooking; not mushy.

300

If you do add fat when preparing your vegetables, monitor it and know exactly how much you are adding per serving. If you are used to a cheese sauce on your vegetables, be sure to try our Low Fat Cheese Sauce in the Sauces section of the recipes.

In the vegetable recipes that follow, we have tried to bring out the natural flavor of the vegetables without adding any fat. We enjoy them, our families enjoy them, and we hope you will too.

Vegetables

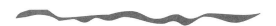

Broccoli

Oriental Vegetables

Spinach

Zucchini

(See Step 25, "Veggie Power," for more ideas.)

301

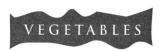
VEGETABLES

Broccoli

2 pounds of broccoli, cleaned
   and cut into 2" pieces

Salt to taste

Optional ingredients:

   Bread crumbs

   Parmesan cheese

   Olive oil spray

302

*If you want to serve the broccoli cold, and want it to
retain the bright green color, after the boiling water is
poured off the broccoli, immediately immerse it in cold
water to stop the cooking process.*

Serves Six

1– Place 4–5 inches of water in a medium-sized pot
   and bring to a boil.

2– Salt the water, and then add the broccoli.

3– Let the water come back to a boil. When the
   broccoli turns bright green, it is ready to serve
   (approximately 2 minutes).

4– Pour off the water and serve.

5– Or, pour off the water and place broccoli in a
   flat serving dish. Lightly spray with olive oil, then
   sprinkle with bread crumbs and Parmesan cheese.

Serving size:

1 cup

Per Serving:

(Nutritional analysis does not include optional ingredients.)
Calories: 60
Grams of carbohydrate: 10
Grams of protein: 4
Grams of fat: .4
2V

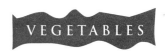

Oriental Vegetables

Vegetable oil spray

2 cups fresh mushrooms, cleaned and sliced

½ yellow onion, skinned and sliced into thin rings

3 green onions, cleaned, cut into 2" lengths

½ cup chicken broth, defatted or nonfat, or vegetable broth

4 cups bean sprouts

4 cups snow peas, washed and stringed

1 bunch asparagus, washed, cut into 4 sections—toss the end section

3 tablespoons lite soy sauce

3 tablespoons oyster sauce

1 teaspoon grated ginger

Salt to taste

Serve as a vegetable dish or over rice as a vegetarian meal, or BBQ some pork chops to serve with them, or sauté 16 ounces of pork strips and add to the vegetable dish.

Serves 12

1– Spray large sauté pan with oil.

2– Sauté the mushrooms and green and yellow onions until brown. Place in a serving bowl.

3– Pour ½ cup broth in the same hot sauté pan and bring to a boil.

4– Add bean sprouts, snow peas and asparagus to hot broth. Sauté and stir until snow peas and asparagus turn bright green. Place these in the serving bowl with the mushroom mixture.

5– Add soy sauce, oyster sauce and ginger to the pan and let these come to a boil. Then pour it over the vegetables in the serving bowl and stir to mix.

303

Serving size:

1 cup

Per Serving:

Calories: 75
Grams of carbohydrate: 12
Grams of protein: 6
Grams of fat: .4
2 ¾V

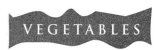
VEGETABLES

Spinach

6 bunches of spinach or
   6 bags of clean spinach

2 cloves of garlic, minced

Salt and pepper to taste

Olive oil spray

304

I usually plan for one bunch/package per person. If some-one extra shows up, you can always add a package of frozen spinach to the fresh. If you are preparing the spinach for later use, cool it down with cold water at step 2, then press out the water. This way you will retain the bright green color.

Serves Six

1– Wash and stem the spinach (be sure to wash the spinach carefully, as it can be quite sandy). Place cleaned spinach in a large pot with 1 inch of boiling water.

2– Cook until limp, then drain and press out most of the water.

3– When well drained, turn spinach onto a cutting board and cut it diagonally one way, then the other. You can serve the spinach as is, or proceed with the rest of the recipe.

4– Spray a sauté pan with a little olive oil and sauté minced garlic until it browns slightly. Add the spinach and cook just long enough to heat and mix thoroughly.

Serving size:

1 cup

Per Serving:

Calories: 63
Grams of carbohydrate: 10
Grams of protein: 4
Grams of fat: .7
2V

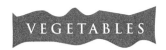
VEGETABLES

Zucchini

2 pounds of zucchini

Salt and pepper to taste

Note:

For a different flavor and texture, you can sauté 3 minced garlic cloves until brown, then add 3 fresh tomatoes, skinned and coarsely chopped. Add the zucchini rounds and simmer until tender, adding 3 basil leaves during the last few minutes.

Serving size:

1 cup

Per Serving:
Calories: 56
Grams of carbohydrate: 10
Grams of protein: 4
Grams of fat: Trace
2V

There are two colors of zucchini. One is very light green and one is dark green. The light green variety has a more delicate flavor and melts in your mouth, so it is worth looking for. It can usually be found at the grocery store in the summer. We grow the light green zucchini in our summer garden for a plentiful supply, and we pick it when it's 3–4 inches long.

Serves Six

1— Wash and cut the zucchini into ¼" rounds.

2— Place zucchini into a pot with 3 inches of boiling, salted water.

3— When the water returns to a boil (after approximately 2 minutes), the zucchini is done. Salt and pepper to taste.

305

Grains & Starches

This category includes all of the breads, beans, pasta, rice, cereal, potatoes
and corn meal. From the Food Pyramid you know that grains and starches should comprise
the majority of your daily food servings. It is important to have some good techniques for
preparing grains and starches so you can incorporate more of them in your meal planning.

Grains and starches are hearty and satisfying foods; they can easily be used in place
of meat as the main dish for a meal. In this recipe section, we have included
many dishes that are meat-free and very satisfying.

306

Grains & Starches

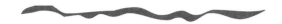

Bulgur Wheat Pilaf

Chunky Potato & Onion Sauté

Corn

Corn Sauté

Creamy Mashed Potatoes

New Potatoes with Baby Onions & Rosemary

Parsley Pasta

Polenta

Risotto with Porcini & Peppers

Skinny French Fries

307

Bulgur Wheat Pilaf

1 cup cracked bulgur wheat

1½ cups boiling water, or nonfat broth

Vegetable oil spray

1 red onion, peeled and chopped

1 yellow onion, peeled and chopped

½ yellow bell pepper, chopped

½ red bell pepper, chopped

2 cloves garlic, cleaned and chopped

2 shallots, cleaned and chopped

1 cup frozen petite peas, thawed

Salt and pepper to taste

308

A nutty, full-flavored dish to have by itself or to accompany a small piece of pork or lamb, surrounded by fresh asparagus.

Serves Eight

1— Place bulgur wheat in a bowl and pour boiling water or broth over it. Let bulgur stand for 45 minutes to 1 hour, until most of the liquid is absorbed. Drain off excess liquid.

2— Spray a large pan with oil and sauté onions, peppers, garlic and shallots until translucent.

3— Add the bulgur to the sauté pan and stir, cooking for 4–5 minutes over medium heat. Excess moisture will cook away so bulgur will become brown and fluffy.

4— Add the peas and cook for 1 minute. Salt and pepper to taste.

Serving size:

1 cup

Per Serving:
Calories: 88
Grams of carbohydrate: 16
Grams of protein: 4.6
Grams of fat: .5
1S, 1V

Chunky Potato & Onion Sauté

6 potatoes, baked

2 red onions, medium size, cleaned

Salt and pepper to taste

1 tablespoon fresh dill
   weed, or 1 teaspoon dried

Olive oil spray

These potatoes are good with any fresh herbs like rosemary, sage or thyme, and are also good plain. When you bake potatoes, bake twice as many and serve the leftovers the next day, chunky style.

Serves Six

1— Cut baked potatoes into ½" cubes, leaving skins on.

2— Cut onions into rings about ¼" thick.

3— Spray sauté pan with oil, then heat to medium-high.

4— Sauté the onion rings until they start to turn translucent and brown.

5— Respray the pan and add the cubed potatoes. Cook until all sides are brown.

6— Sprinkle with fresh or dried dill weed and heat thoroughly before serving.

309

Serving size:

¾ cup

Per Serving:
Calories: 178
Grams of carbohydrate: 33
Grams of protein: 5
Grams of fat: 2.3
2S, ½V

Corn

6 ears of corn, husked, washed and broken in half

2 tablespoons of lite butter

2 tablespoons water

Salt and pepper to taste

310

I like to fix twice as much corn as the recipe calls for, so I can sauté the extra kernels with onion and fresh red and yellow bell peppers the next night.

This technique of melting butter and water on a plate and then rolling the corn in it gives you good coverage with less fat.

Serves Six

1– Start a large pot of water boiling.

2– Immerse the corn in the water and bring back to a boil. Corn is done when water comes back to a boil.

3– Melt the butter and 2 tablespoons of water on a flat plate in the microwave oven for approximately 1 minute (microwave cooking times vary).

4– Roll the corn in the butter mixture, then salt and pepper to taste, or eat the corn plain.

Serving size:

1 ear of corn

Per Serving:

Calories: 172
Grams of carbohydrate: 30
Grams of protein: 4
Grams of fat: 4
2S, ½Fa

Corn Sauté

6 ears of corn, cleaned and boiled

Vegetable oil spray

1 yellow or red onion, cut into fine strips

½ red bell pepper, cut into fine strips

½ yellow bell pepper, cut into fine strips

1 clove of garlic, minced

If you're in a hurry, use frozen corn or frozen peas as a substitute for fresh corn. The bell peppers and yellow or red onion make a great color and flavor combination with these two starches.

Serves Six

1— Remove the cooked corn from the ear with a knife.

2— Sauté the onion in a medium pan lightly sprayed with oil until it becomes translucent.

3— Add the red and yellow peppers and the garlic. Sauté until the peppers are tender and sweet.

4— Add the corn kernels and cook just enough to heat the corn thoroughly, then serve.

311

Serving size:

¾ cup

Per Serving:

Calories: 211
Grams of carbohydrate: 40
Grams of protein: 6.6
Grams of fat: 2.8
2S, 1½V

Creamy Mashed Potatoes

8 red new potatoes,
medium to large size

¼ cup nonfat sour cream

¼ cup skim evaporated milk

¼ cup lite butter or whipped
butter (6 grams of fat per
tablespoon) or nonfat margarine

Salt and pepper to taste

Flavor options:

1 tablespoon horseradish

2 cloves of garlic, browned and
mashed

4 tablespoons red onion, grated

Roasted red bell pepper, chopped

Normally, I don't add butter or margarine to food, but in mashed potatoes I like a little butter for flavor.

Serves Six

1— Clean and cut each potato (unpeeled) into six pieces and place into boiling, salted water.

2— Boil until potatoes are tender.

3— Drain water from potatoes.

4— Blend potatoes with an electric mixer until almost smooth, then add remaining ingredients and blend until smooth.

5— Salt and pepper to taste.

312

Serving size:

1 cup

Per Serving:

Calories: 150
Grams of carbohydrate: 22
Grams of protein: 4
Grams of fat: 5
1½S, ¾Fa

New Potatoes with Baby Onions & Rosemary

30 red new potatoes, small size

20 1" pearl onions, skinned

Olive oil spray

6 sprigs of fresh rosemary

Dash of white wine or
  chicken broth, defatted
  or nonfat, or vegetable broth

Salt, pepper and garlic powder
  to taste

Serving size:

1 cup or 6 pieces

Per Serving:

Calories: 116
Grams of carbohydrate: 21
Grams of protein: 3.5
Grams of fat: 2
1½S, ¼V

The infusion of the rosemary while roasting with the potatoes and onions has an inticing aroma. The potatoes and onions will be toasty brown on the outside and tender and sweet inside. I like to buy the peewee size that is about 1–1½" in diameter.

Serves Eight

1– Preheat oven to 375°.

2– Spray oil into glass or metal roasting pan, just enough to coat the pan.

3– Place your cleaned red potatoes, onions, and stripped leaves of rosemary in a bowl, and spray with olive oil to coat.

4– Salt, pepper and garlic powder the potatoes to taste.

5– Place potatoes and onions in the roasting pan.

6– Several times during the cooking, loosen potatoes from the pan and turn them over. Spray with oil if necessary. Add a little broth or wine to the bottom of the pan near the end of the cooking time for added moisture and flavor.

7– Bake for 1–1½ hours, until done.

313

Parsley Pasta

16–18 ounces dry pasta, like penne, angel hair or linguine

1 tablespoon olive oil

2 tablespoons vegetable broth, or nonfat chicken or beef broth

2 tablespoons parsley or basil, cleaned and chopped fine

Salt and pepper to taste

Everyone is talking about cooking pasta al dente. Literally, this translates as "to the tooth." Practically, it refers to pasta that is cooked just to the point where it loses the taste of flour and is chewy in texture.

Serves Eight

1– Bring a large pot of water to a boil and lightly salt.

2– Add pasta to boiling water and cook al dente (depending on the type of pasta, 7–11 minutes).

3– Heat oil and broth in a microwave oven for 1 minute.

4– Drain pasta and place in a large bowl. Add heated oil and broth, and chopped parsley or basil. Stir to mix.

5– Salt and pepper to taste.

314

Serving size:

1 cup

Per Serving:

Calories: 173
Grams of carbohydrate: 30
Grams of protein: 4
Grams of fat: 3.8
2S, ¼Fa

Polenta

Polenta is a traditional Italian dish, used much the same way rice is used in Chinese cooking. It can be combined with vegetables and sauces for one-dish meals, or topped with cheese for added flavor. Use it as you would use rice.

We always make twice as much as we want because it's great the next day. You can make half the recipe soft polenta and pour the other half onto an oiled baking sheet and chill until firm. It can then be cut into shapes for baking, frying or grilling.

Select a large, heavy pot so when the polenta boils it won't stick to the pan and it won't boil over onto the stove.

315

Serves Eight

8 cups cold water

2 cups coarse cornmeal

1– Bring water to a boil in a large pot.

2– Pour polenta (cornmeal) into the boiling water in a slow, steady stream, stirring constantly so no lumps form.

3– Reduce temperature so you get a minimal, continuous boil. Stir every few minutes to reduce sticking.

4– The polenta is done when it is soft on the tongue and not grainy in texture, about 20 minutes. If you want a softer polenta, add more water.

Serving size:

1 cup

Per Serving:

Calories: 110
Grams of carbohydrate: 22.5
Grams of protein: 2.8
Grams of fat: 1
1½S

Risotto with Porcini & Peppers

½ cup dried Porcini mushrooms, soaked and diced medium

1½ cups boiling hot water

1 cup parsley leaves

2 yellow onions, quartered

1 tablespoon olive oil

2 cups Arborio rice

1 red bell pepper, cleaned and cut into ¼" strips

1 yellow bell pepper, cleaned and cut into ¼" strips

5–6 cups chicken broth, defatted or nonfat, or vegetable broth

¼ cup Parmesan cheese

Salt and pepper to taste

316

Arborio rice is grown in the northern part of Italy. It has a hardness to the center of the grain, and should be served al dente (chewy).

Serves Eight

1– Soak dried mushrooms in 1½ cups boiling hot water for 30 minutes. Remove mushrooms from water. Strain the mushroom water through a cheesecloth and set aside. Dice mushrooms to a medium chop.

2– Place parsley and onions in a food processor and chop fine.

3– In a large sauté pan, heat oil and sauté onions and parsley until translucent.

4– Add the rice and stir occasionally, until it starts to turn translucent; about 5 minutes.

5– Add the peppers, mushrooms and the mushroom water to the pan.

6– Heat the broth and add hot broth to the pan, a cupful at a time, while stirring constantly. Allow the rice to absorb the broth before adding more. This process should take 15–20 minutes. You may not need all of the broth.

7– When rice is al dente (chewy in texture), it is done. To serve, sprinkle with Parmesan cheese and salt and pepper to taste.

Serving size:

1 cup

Per Serving:

Calories: 188
Grams of carbohydrate: 29
Grams of protein: 9
Grams of fat: 3.7
2S, 1V, ¼Fa

Skinny French Fries

This recipe is one of our students' favorites. The technique of measuring oil into a Ziploc bag to coat potatoes can be used for other starches and vegetable recipes where you want a crisp fried flavor. There are several French fry cutters on the market which save time and give you an even cut. If you serve French fries often, you may be able to justify the cost.

8 russet potatoes, cleaned

1 tablespoon oil

Salt to taste

Vegetable oil spray

Serves Eight

1— Preheat oven to 450°.

2— If you are not using a French fry cutter, cut each potato in half. Cut each half into ¼" strips.

3— Place potato strips into a quart plastic Ziploc bag with the oil and shake to coat.

4— Spray 2 cookie sheets with oil and spread potatoes evenly onto them. It is very important to keep them spread apart (I don't even let them touch).

5— Bake for 45–55 minutes or until crispy and brown. Turn occasionally so they brown all over and don't stick to the pan. Salt and serve.

317

Serving size:

1 potato

Per Serving:

Calories: 133
Grams of carbohydrate: 22.5
Grams of protein: 3
Grams of fat: 3.4
1½S, ½Fa

Sauces

Sauces are to cooking what melodies are to songs—but, unfortunately, many of them are traditionally high in fat. In the following recipes, you'll find several basic, low fat alternatives that can be used over pasta, as a Cioppino or as the base for a stew.

A good low fat sauce we use frequently is Béchamel Sauce. This is a creamy white sauce that goes well with many different dishes. It can be used in place of a heavy cream sauce on pasta, or on vegetables as an alternative to cheese. Its flavor can easily be altered to suit your recipe by adding fresh herbs, low fat cheese or seasonings such as nutmeg.

Our Yogurt Cheese recipe is also quite versatile. It can be used in place of a cream spread or served as a dip for fresh vegetables or even used in a soup to add a creamy texture and taste.

318

Sauces

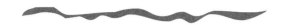

Basic White Sauce (Sauce Béchamel)
Giovanna's Basic Sauce
Low Fat Cheese Sauce
Pasta with Pesto (Original Recipe)
Pasta with Pestolino
Teresa's Tomato Sauce
Tomato Cran Salsa
Tomato Sauce Semplice
Yogurt Cheese Sauce

319

Basic White Sauce (Sauce Béchamel)

2 tablespoons butter

2 tablespoons flour

1 cup nonfat milk

Salt, white ground pepper and
   nutmeg to taste

Serves Six

320

Serving size:

3 tablespoons

Per Serving:
Calories: 74
Grams of carbohydrate: 4.2
Grams of protein: 1.6
Grams of fat: 5
¼D, 1Fa

*This sauce is a good substitute for alfredo sauce, which has
33 grams of fat per serving (compared with 5 grams here).
It's great with white albacore tuna or leftover chicken and
frozen peas and green onions for color. Or, try adding ¼
pound prosciutto, cut in thin strips, with peas, green onions
and parsley, served over pasta.*

For the experienced cook:

1— Melt butter in saucepan over low heat. Blend in
flour; it's good if the flour cooks for 5 to 10 seconds.

2— Add milk slowly while using a whisk. Cook over a
medium heat, stirring constantly until mixture
thickens and bubbles.

3— Add salt, ground white pepper and freshly ground
nutmeg to taste.

For the inexperienced cook:

1— Melt butter in saucepan over low heat. When melted,
turn pan off and set aside.

2— Place the flour in a small bowl and add enough milk
to make a paste. Gradually add the remaining milk,
stirring, until the mixture is smooth.

3— Return the saucepan with butter to the stove over
low heat. Add the flour mixture to the butter and stir
until sauce thickens.

4— Add salt, pepper and nutmeg to taste.

Giovanna's Basic Sauce

1 yellow onion, cleaned
   and quartered

4 cloves of garlic, cleaned

2 shallots, cleaned

2 stalks celery, cleaned and cut
   into 4 pieces

1 carrot, cut into 4 pieces

1 cup parsley, cleaned

1½ tablespoons
   butter or oil

½ cup wine or ½ cup
   chicken broth, defatted or
   nonfat, or vegetable broth

1 28-ounce can whole, peeled
   tomatoes

Salt and pepper to taste

Variations:

Fresh mushrooms

Chopped leeks

Sautéed baby onions

Fresh herbs
   (sage, thyme or rosemary)

This sauce is a mainstay. You can add a variety of other ingredients to make it more complex—whatever is in the "fridge" or pantry. After making the sauce you can add a variety of fish and cook until the fish is done to make a Cioppino. Turn this sauce into a stew by adding beef or lamb and simmering on low until the meat is tender. Of course, it's also good on pasta!

Serves 6-8

1— Place the onions, garlic, shallots, celery, carrots and parsley in food processor and pulse 20 times or until medium fine.

2— In a heavy saucepan heat the butter or oil and sauté the above ingredients from the food processor until brown and translucent.

3— Add the wine or broth to deglaze the pan. The alcohol will burn off in a few minutes so only the sweet, rich, wine grape flavor remains.

4— Add the whole tomatoes (cut into pieces), or 6 fresh tomatoes, peeled, seeded and diced, and cook until flavors blend.

321

Serving size:

½ cup sauce

Per Serving:

Calories: 73
Grams of carbohydrate: 8
Grams of protein: 3
Grams of fat: 3.2
1V, ½Fa

Low Fat Cheese Sauce

2 tablespoons lite butter

2 tablespoons flour

1½ cups nonfat milk

½ cup fat free sharp cheddar cheese, grated (Alpine Lace makes a good variety)

2 tablespoons dry white wine

Salt and pepper to taste

Some people want to have a little sauce on whatever they eat, including vegetables. This cheese sauce will give you a rich cheese flavor with very little fat.

Yield: 2 cups

1– Melt butter in medium saucepan over low heat.

2– Sprinkle flour over melted butter and stir to make a roux.

3– Slowly whisk in milk and stir until roux is completely incorporated into milk.

4– Continue stirring over medium heat until mixture is thick and bubbly.

5– Add cheese, onion and wine and stir until cheese melts.

6– Remove from heat. Salt and pepper to taste.

322

Serving size:
2 tablespoons

Per Serving:
Calories: 58
Grams of carbohydrate: 4.8
Grams of protein: 5.8
Grams of fat: 1.8
¼D, ½P, ¼Fa

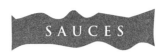

SAUCES

Pasta with Pesto (Original Recipe)

1 colander of basil (10" x 5") cleaned, stemmed and blanched

4 cloves fresh garlic

1 cup olive oil

6 ounces Parmesan cheese

¾ cup butter, softened to room temperature

¼ cup heavy whipping cream

6 pounds of pasta

We serve Pasta with Pesto at almost every big family gathering we have. If it's balanced correctly between the fresh basil, oil, garlic and cheese it is yummy but very high in fat. I modified this recipe on the next page and called it "Pasta with Pestolino" to give you a more "lino" choice.

Yield: 2 ½ cups

1– Blanch basil for 30 seconds in boiling water. Drain the leaves and press out extra water from them.

2– Place basil in a food processor, add garlic and process until well chopped.

3– With processor running, slowly add olive oil and Parmesan cheese, reserving one ounce of the cheese to sprinkle on top of the pasta with pesto.

4– Slowly add butter and heavy whipping cream to processor.

5– Boil pasta, drain and pour into a large bowl. Add pesto sauce from processor to pasta and toss until blended. This sauce is enough for 6 pounds of pasta.

NOTE:

1– *Sprinkle some Parmesan cheese and pine nuts on top of the Pasta with Pesto before serving.*

2– *If you place the finished Pasta with Pesto in a warm pot and cover, it will stay warm for 30–40 minutes.*

323

Serving size:
1 tablespoon

Per Serving:
(sauce only)
Calories: 108
Grams of carbohydrates: .2
Grams of protein: .9
Grams of fat: 11.5
2¼Fa

Pasta with Pestolino

1½ cups lightly packed basil leaves, cleaned and stemmed

1–3 garlic cloves, cleaned*

½ cup lite butter

¼ cup nonfat vanilla ice cream

⅛ cup olive oil

¼ cup Parmesan cheese

⅛ cup chicken broth, defatted or nonfat, or vegetable broth

1 teaspoon salt

12 ounces pasta, dried or fresh

Garlic can be very powerful or weak. Start with one clove. You can always add more to your taste.

324

This is a lighter version of the original Pasta with Pesto recipe. Into the boiling pasta water I like to throw 2 or 3 small light green zucchini cut into small slices or 2 red new potatoes sliced thin. It adds an interesting contrast to the pesto.

Yield: 2 cups

1— Blanch basil leaves in boiling water for 30 seconds. Drain the leaves and press excess water from them.

2— Place basil, butter and garlic in a food processor. Process until well blended.

3— Add the next five ingredients and process until smooth. Taste to see if you need more garlic.

4— Boil pasta in salted water until al dente (chewy), drain and pour into a large bowl. Add the pestolino and toss until blended.

5— If you prepare the pestolino ahead, cover it and refrigerate until ready to use. Never heat the pesto sauce. When ready to serve, pour hot pasta into a warmed bowl, add the pesto sauce and toss.

Serving size: 1 tablespoon

Note: ½ cup sauce covers one 12-ounce package of noodles, which makes 8 cups when cooked.

Per Serving:

	(Sauce Only) Original Recipe	(Sauce Only) Modified Recipe
Calories:	108	43
Grams of carbohydrate:	0.2	.8
Grams of protein:	0.9	2
Grams of fat:	**11.5**	**3.5**

¾Fa

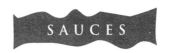

SAUCES

Teresa's Tomato Sauce

3 tomatoes, vine-ripe
(the riper the tomato, the
sweeter the sauce)

1 cup tomato sauce

2 tablespoons olive oil

4 cloves garlic, cleaned
and chopped fine

6 sprigs basil

Teresa is an incredible Italian cook. After her honeymoon of eight days in 1934, her husband brought her home to the farm. The male cook, seeing a woman come into the house, quit, and the next day she cooked for twelve men and did their washing and ironing. These were the days when you killed your own chickens, three at once to save time. It was not the push-button, micro-age.

Teresa's techniques give food a delicate texture, beautiful color and fabulous flavor.

Serves Six

1— Skin the tomatoes. You can use two methods. Either sear tomatoes on all sides over a gas stove by holding them over the fire with a long fork or tongs, or you can place the tomatoes in a pot of boiling water for 1 minute.

325

2— Cut the tomatoes into rough chunks and put in a small pot to cook down until soft, 10–15 minutes. Add 1 cup of tomato sauce to fresh tomatoes.

3— While tomatoes are cooking, finely chop 3 cloves of garlic and sauté them in 2 tablespoons of oil, being careful not to burn them.

4— Put the cooked tomatoes through a food mill. This eliminates the seeds.

Serving size:
⅓ cup sauce

Per Serving:
Calories: 90
Grams of carbohydrates: 7.5
Grams of protein: 3
Grams of fat: 5
1V, 1Fa

5— Return the tomatoes to the pot and add the browned garlic. Turn up the fire to medium and add your cleaned, fresh basil to this mixture.

6— Cook another 5 minutes on low to blend the flavors and add salt and ground pepper to taste. Also, a small pinch of sugar will heighten the flavors. Serve over pasta or gnocchi.

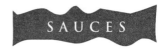

SAUCES

Tomato Cran Salsa

1 bag fresh cranberries

1 cup sugar

½ cup red onions, diced

2 Serrano chiles, seeded and minced

¼ cup cilantro, cleaned, stemmed and chopped

2 tomatoes, vine-ripe, skinned, and chopped medium fine

Note: You can substitute a can of whole cranberries, when cranberries are not in season. When you do this, omit the sugar, but add the rest of the ingredients. You can also eliminate the tomatoes for a slightly different flavor.

326

This is a wonderful, tongue-tantalizing salsa. It's great on a baguette with grilled chicken, or a fresh piece of salmon.

Serves Six

1— Wash cranberries and combine with sugar in a microwave-safe container.

2— Cover and microwave on high for 4 minutes.

3— Stir. Cook 4 more minutes on high.

4— When cool, stir in remaining ingredients.

Serving size:

½ cup

Per Serving:
Calories: 82
Grams of carbohydrates: 20
Grams of protein: .5
Grams of fat: 0
¼V, ¼Fa (sugar)

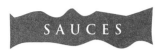
SAUCES

Tomato Sauce Semplice

¼–½ cup combination of fresh thyme, basil and parsley, cleaned and stemmed

2 cloves garlic, cleaned

2 shallots, cleaned

1 yellow onion, cleaned and quartered

2 tablespoons olive oil (1 tablespoon works, and would cut the fat per serving in half)

½ cup wine or chicken broth, defatted or nonfat, or vegetable broth

6 large, fresh tomatoes, peeled, seeded and chopped

Salt and pepper to taste

If you're in a hurry, open a 28-ounce can of whole, peeled plum tomatoes and cut them into pieces or open a 28-ounce can of whole ground tomatoes. Use these instead of fresh tomatoes. Serve this sauce over your favorite pasta or fish. Or serve it over a dish of polenta, sprinkling some low fat grated cheese over the top and broiling until it melts.

Serves 12

1– Place herbs in food processor and chop fine.

2– Add the garlic, shallots and onions and pulse 20 times until chopped medium fine.

3– In a medium saucepan add olive oil and heat to high. Add your mixture from the food processor and sauté until brown and translucent.

4– Deglaze the pan with the wine or broth, then turn off heat.

5– Sear whole tomatoes over a gas burner or place them in boiling water for 1 minute. Peel and deseed. Coarsely chop tomatoes, add to saucepan and continue heating on high for 3–5 minutes until blended.

327

Serving size:

½ cup

Per Serving:
Calories: 64
Grams of carbohydrate: 7
Grams of protein: 2.8
Grams of fat: 2.8
1V, ½Fa

Yogurt Cheese Sauce

8 ounces nonfat plain yogurt without gelatin, cornstarch or other
thickeners (pectin is all right)

Equipment needed:

Yogurt strainer

Cheesecloth or other fine mesh
strainer, or small holes cut in the
bottom of the yogurt carton

2-cup glass measuring cup

*Yogurt cheese is a nonfat, creamy substance that can be
substituted in recipes that call for cream or mayonnaise.
Some yogurt brands that work for this recipe are
Continental and Dannon Light.*

Yield: ½ cup

1— Place yogurt in cheesecloth or other strainer on top
of 2-cup glass measuring cup and put in refrigerator
overnight. The longer it's in the refrigerator, the
more it will drain.

2— You will have a thick yogurt "cheese" or "cream"
in the strainer and a liquid in the cup. Throw the
liquid out.

3— Use this "cream" like a mayonnaise or sour cream,
or use it to make low fat or nonfat dips, to make a
soup creamy or, diluted, to substitute for cream in a
recipe.

Serving size:

½ cup

Per Serving:
Calories: 60
Grams of carbohydrate: 9
Grams of protein: 6
Grams of fat: 0
¾D

328

Entrees

Dinner is often the only time a family can sit down together and enjoy a good meal. It's important to have a wide repertoire of recipes that all family members can enjoy, so that dinner does not become repetitive and boring. One way to assure variety is to refer to Step 21 for help with menu planning and shopping. Planning ahead can eliminate some stress at dinner time!

In this recipe section, we have tried to include a wide variety of recipes, so that there is something for everyone. Each of these recipes can be modified to suit your family's particular tastes. For example, in our Chicken, Herb & Mushroom Sauté, you can substitute another type of meat for the chicken and other vegetables for the mushrooms. The trick is to learn the cooking techniques and how to substitute foods. Remember, what we are trying to do is simply cut the fat without giving up the flavor or the dishes we love.

330

Entrees

Chicken, Herb & Mushroom Sauté
Enchajitas
Fish Stew over Polenta
Italian Fried Chicken
Pasta Tuna Béchamel
Roast with Carrots, Onions & Potatoes
Stuffed Pork Roast
Swiss Chicken

331

Chicken, Herb & Mushroom Sauté

6 skinless chicken breast halves

4 stems each of rosemary, sage and thyme, cleaned and stemmed

1 pound fresh mushrooms

1 tablespoon olive oil

Olive oil spray

½ cup wine

½ cup chicken broth, defatted or nonfat

Salt, pepper, garlic powder to taste

Cornstarch as needed

332

This is a delicious, fast dinner that is good with low fat mashed potatoes and a fresh vegetable. You can substitute a can of mushrooms for the fresh, but it won't taste as good.

Serves Six

1— Cut chicken breasts into three diagonal pieces. Sprinkle with salt, pepper and garlic powder to taste on all sides.

2— Put rosemary, sage and thyme leaves in a food processor and pulse until fine. Cover chicken pieces with the finely chopped herbs.

3— Clean mushrooms and slice.

4— Heat oil and brown chicken on both sides. Remove to another dish.

5— Spray pan with olive oil and sauté sliced mushrooms.

6— Add chicken back to the pan and deglaze the pan with the wine or chicken broth.

7— If you want more sauce, add more wine or broth. For a thicker sauce, add 1 tablespoon of cornstarch to the wine or broth before adding it to the pan.

Serving size:
1 chicken breast

Per Serving:
Calories: 173
Grams of carbohydrate: 3.3
Grams of protein: 23
Grams of fat: 5.5
¼V, 3P, ½Fa

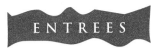

Enchajitas

1 red onion, cleaned and sliced in long slivers

1 yellow onion, cleaned and sliced in long slivers

1 red bell pepper, cleaned and sliced in long slivers

1 yellow bell pepper, cleaned and sliced in long slivers

4 boneless chicken breasts, cut on the diagonal into ¼" strips

1 4-ounce can green chiles, diced

5 ounces low fat Mozzarella cheese, grated

1 package of 12 tortillas, with 1 gram of fat per tortilla

2 10-ounce cans enchilada sauce— canned or homemade (a good salsa could be substituted or mixed with enchilada sauce)

Vegetable oil spray

Salt, pepper and garlic powder to taste

One afternoon, debating in my head which Mexican dish to have—enchiladas or fajitas—I decided to make my own interpretation of the best of both. It is fajita ingredients baked like an enchilada.

Serves Six

1— Spray a medium sauté pan with vegetable oil and add red and yellow onions and red and yellow bell peppers. Sauté until onions start to turn color and bell peppers get a little color. Salt to taste.

2— Remove onions and peppers to a bowl and respray the pan with oil. Add strips of chicken breast seasoned with garlic powder and salt and pepper to taste. Sauté a few minutes until done and remove chicken to the bowl of onions and peppers.

3— Add the can of green chiles and 4 ounces of the Mozzarella to the same bowl and mix, leaving 1 ounce of Mozzarella to put on top of the finished Enchajitas.

4— Respray the same pan and cook each tortilla on both sides, then add a handful of the mixture to each tortilla. Roll up and place in a sprayed 9" x 12" oven-proof dish.

5— Pour your favorite enchilada sauce on top of the 12 filled tortillas and sprinkle remaining Mozzarella on top.

6— Heat for 20–25 minutes at 350°.

333

Serving size:
2 filled tortillas

Per Serving:
Calories: 355
Grams of carbohydrate: 43
Grams of protein: 26
Grams of fat: 7.6
2S, 2V, 3P

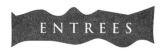

Fish Stew over Polenta

Giovanna's Basic Sauce
  (see recipe on page 321)

1 package Pheasant brand
  polenta

8 cups of water

8-ounce piece of sea bass or filet of
  sole, cut into small pieces

16 clams, washed and brushed

16 mussels, washed and brushed

38–40 medium shrimp (can be
  bought cleaned and frozen)

1½ pounds scallops, large ones cut
  in quarters

Salt and pepper to taste

Variations: Add your favorite shell-
fish in season. You can also add
clam juice and canned clams.

334

Serving size:
1 cup polenta with 1 cup fish stew

Per Serving:
Calories: 322
Grams of carbohydrate: 34
Grams of protein: 28
Grams of fat: 6.5
2S, ½V, 3P, ¼Fa

This is one of my favorite winter dishes. I serve it with a green salad and warmed bread.

Serves 6–8

1— Follow directions for Giovanna's Basic Sauce.

2— Put 8 cups of water in a pot and when it boils add 2 cups of polenta very slowly. Keep stirring. Add salt to taste. Stir for approximately 20 minutes until it is smooth—not grainy to taste. Leave out any butter it tells you to add on the package. If the polenta gets hard before the stew is ready, add a little water (½ cup). Stir and reheat.

3— Add sea bass to Giovanna's sauce and cook on medium heat for five minutes or until fish disintegrates.

4— Add clams and mussels and cook until they open. Add shrimp and scallops. Cook until shrimp turns orange.

5— Serve polenta on plate with a scoop of fish stew on top.

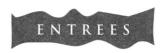

Italian Fried Chicken

6 skinless chicken breast halves

1 carton egg substitute

1 cup flour

1 lemon, cut into 6 pieces

1 teaspoon salt

½ teaspoon pepper

1 teaspoon garlic powder

Olive oil spray

Variations: This can be done with turkey or pork very successfully.

Our children and grandchildren love this with a squeeze of lemon and sometimes ketchup.

Serves Six

1— Butterfly the chicken breast into two pieces, lengthwise, like cutting open a roll for a sandwich. You need a sharp knife to do this evenly, and the chicken needs to be cold.

2— Put egg substitute into a pie dish and sprinkle with salt, pepper and garlic powder. Stir this mixture with a fork.

3— Put chicken breasts into the egg mixture.

4— Put flour in another pie dish.

5— Remove one breast at a time, dip into the flour to coat, and then shake off excess flour.

6— When all the chicken pieces are coated with flour, spray a sauté pan with olive oil and brown the pieces on both sides. You will need to use the oil spray to coat the second side for a nice browning.

335

Serving size:

2 pieces

Per Serving:

Calories: 331
Grams of carbohydrate: 19
Grams of protein: 44
Grams of fat: 8.8
1S, 16P, ½Fa

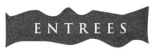

Pasta Tuna Béchamel

1 recipe Basic White Sauce
(see recipe on page 322)

1 can (12¼ ounce) white
albacore tuna in water, drained

2 tablespoons nonfat
sour cream

1 package of frozen petite peas

4 green onions, sliced

1 package of noodles without
eggs—your choice of shells,
linguine, etc.

Salt and pepper

Variations: This can be cooked
with shrimp, chicken or turkey.

*My mom used to have tuna in cream sauce with peas
ready when she and Dad went out, which was not very
often. This is a modern version of that recipe. We cut the
fat (Mom used a whole cube of butter) and put the
béchamel sauce on pasta instead of toast.*

Serves Six

1— Make one recipe of Basic White Sauce.

2— Add tuna and nonfat sour cream to the white sauce
and stir over high heat until blended. Add package
of peas and green onions and cook to blend.

3— Cook pasta in a large pot of boiling, salted water
until al dente (chewy). Drain.

4— Pour pasta immediately into warm sauce and serve
from the pan.

336

Serving size:
2 cups

Per Serving:
Calories: 398
Grams of carbohydrate: 53
Grams of protein: 24
Grams of fat: 10
3S, 1V, ¼D, 2P, 1Fa

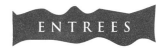

ENTREES

Roast with Carrots, Onions & Potatoes

4–5 pound tenderloin pork roast

3 garlic cloves, cleaned and cut into 4 slices per clove

6 sprigs fresh rosemary

4 carrots, cleaned and cut into 1" slices

1 basket of small onions, cleaned and left whole

8 russet potatoes

Salt, pepper and garlic powder to taste

Olive oil spray

Serves Six

Serving size:
⅙ of roast with vegetables

Per Serving:
Calories: 483
Grams of carbohydrate: 35
Grams of protein: 49
Grams of fat: 14.6
2S, 1V, 6P, 1Fa

There's nothing simpler to make than a roast and potatoes for the family on a Friday and then have leftovers for Saturday or Sunday. This is a way to make it tasty and cut the fat.

1— Preheat oven to 350°. Sprinkle salt, pepper and garlic powder to taste on the roast.

2— Make 12 holes in different places on the roast and poke the garlic pieces into the holes.

3— Poke the rosemary under the string that comes wrapped around the roast and into creases of the folded meat.

4— Place the carrots, onions and potatoes into a bowl, sprinkle with salt, pepper and garlic powder to taste, and then spray vegetables with oil.

5— Spray the roasting pan with oil, add roast, then place the vegetables around the roast. Place roast in pre-heated oven.

6— After 30 minutes, turn the potatoes, carrots and onions and respray with oil. After 15 more minutes repeat turning and spraying.

7— Cook for 1 hour longer and serve. Total time to cook should be 1½–1¾ hours. Divide the roast and vegetables into six equal portions.

337

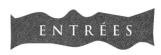
ENTRÉES

Stuffed Pork Roast

2½ pounds pork tenderloin, trimmed of fat and membrane

Salt, pepper and garlic powder to taste

2 small apples, chopped

1 cup soft bread crumbs

½ cup chopped celery

4 tablespoons raisins

4 tablespoons walnuts, chopped

2 green onions, sliced

4 tablespoons apple juice

Sauce for roast:

1 cup apple juice

3 teaspoons cornstarch

⅛ teaspoon ground cinnamon

Fresh ground nutmeg to taste

2–3 tablespoons apricot jam, the all-fruit variety

338

Serving size:
2 slices with sauce

Per Serving:
Calories: 208
Grams of carbohydrate: 17
Grams of protein: 20
Grams of fat: 6
½S, ¼Fr, 3P

This dish gives a pretty presentation and can be made ahead of time. Each loin cuts into six or seven pieces. When you buy the tenderloin it will be two pieces tied together. Cut the string and separate.

Serves Eight

1— To butterfly the tenderloin, make a cut lengthwise and stop within ½" of the other side (like cutting a french roll in half but keeping a hinge). Repeat this procedure for the other piece.

2— Cover tenderloin with plastic wrap and pound with a meat mallet to ½" thickness. Season with salt, pepper and garlic powder to taste.

3— For the stuffing, place next six ingredients in a bowl and moisten with 2 tablespoons of apple juice.

4— Spread stuffing over tenderloins. Roll up from the narrow side and tie with string to secure. Brush tenderloins with 2 tablespoons of apple juice.

5— Place tenderloins in a roasting pan in a preheated 350° oven for 1¼ hours or until done. Take roast out of pan and place on platter in warm spot.

6— In the roasting pan, stir together 1 cup apple juice, cornstarch, cinnamon and nutmeg. Also add 2 or 3 tablespoons of apricot jam. Cook and stir over medium heat until thickened. Serve over tenderloins.

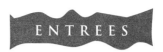
ENTREES

Swiss Chicken

6 boneless, skinned chicken breasts

6 slices Alpine brand Swiss cheese, or any nonfat variety

Olive oil spray

2 cups sliced mushrooms

1 can 97% fat-free cream of mushroom soup

1 cup nonfat sour cream

½ cup sherry or ½ cup dry white wine

Salt, pepper, garlic powder and paprika to taste

Serving size:

1 breast with sauce

Per Serving:
Calories: 203
Grams of carbohydrate: 9
Grams of protein: 32
Grams of fat: 4.3
½V, 4P

This is a simple, fast recipe for when you're in a hurry. You can even skip sautéing the mushrooms and pour all the ingredients on top of the chicken when pushed for time.

Serves Six

1— Preheat oven to 350°. Place chicken breasts in a 2-quart baking dish; season with salt, pepper and garlic powder to taste.

2— Cover breasts with cheese.

3— Sauté sliced mushrooms in a sauté pan sprayed with oil.

4— Deglaze pan of sautéed mushrooms with ½ cup sherry or white wine.

5— Pour soup and nonfat sour cream in with the mushrooms and the wine. Warm through, then pour this mixture over the chicken and cheese.

6— Sprinkle with paprika.

7— Bake uncovered at 350° for 45–50 minutes.

339

Desserts

Desserts, desserts, desserts!
They are so tempting at the bakery, so enticing at
a restaurant, so seductive on a plate, and so full of sugar and fat!

Yes, we know that the majority of our food intake should come from the bottom
of the Food Pyramid, but what our body doesn't need, out mouths and tummies want!
The key is not to deprive yourself of desserts, but to discipline yourself about them.

Many desserts can be prepared in a low fat way, and we have included enough of them
in this section to lure you away from the high fat ones and tempt you with low fat alternatives.
Don't make traditional desserts a habit. Do treat yourself to an occasional dessert,
and when you do, make a smart choice.

340

Desserts

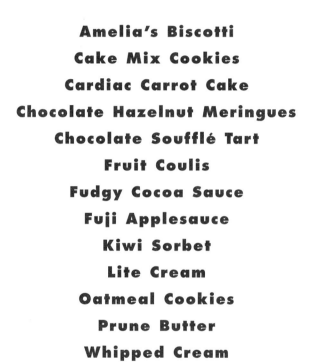

341

DESSERTS

Amelia's Biscotti

Low fat ingredients:
Vegetable oil spray

1 cup whole almonds

4 cups flour

1½ cups sugar

3 teaspoons baking powder

½ cup lite butter, melted

2 egg whites

1¼ cup egg substitute

Original ingredients:
2 cups almonds

3 cups flour

1½ cups sugar

3 teaspoons baking powder

½ cup butter, melted

3 whole eggs

3 egg whites

342

Serving size:
1 Biscotti

Per Serving:

	Original	Low Fat
Calories:	49	32
Grams of carbohydrate:	5.5	6
Grams of protein:	1	1
Grams of fat:	**2.3**	**0.5**

½S

Compare the low fat ingredients to the original ingredients and you will see how to make changes in your favorite recipes. You can make chocolate biscotti by adding ½ cup Dutch process cocoa.

Yield: 10 dozen

1— Preheat oven to 350° and prepare two large cookie sheets with vegetable oil.

2— Spread almonds onto small, ungreased pan and bake at 350° for 8 minutes.

3— Sift together flour, sugar and baking powder and add the toasted almonds.

4— Beat egg whites until frothy, and set aside.

5— Combine melted butter and egg substitute with a fork in a small bowl.

6— Put flour mixture on a board (or leave in a bowl) and make a well in the center. In the well put the combined melted butter and egg substitute.

7— Work eggs and butter into the flour until it forms a ball. Divide ball into eight smaller balls. Roll each ball into dough sticks the length of a cookie sheet, pat down, and brush with beaten egg whites.

8— Bake at 350° for 20–30 minutes until golden brown. Remove from the oven and remove sticks from cookie tray. Cut sticks into ½" angular pieces and return to tray. Turn cookies on sides and bake again at 300° for 5–10 minutes or until crispy.

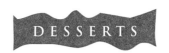

DESSERTS

Cake Mix Cookies

1 box "lite" cake mix (lemon, chocolate or white)

½ cup egg substitute

3 tablespoons nonfat milk

2 tablespoons canola oil

½ cup mini chocolate chips *(optional)*

Vegetable oil spray

Cake mix cookies are never as good as homemade but they are a fun starter recipe for kids, and a way to save time and cleanup.

Yield: 4 dozen

1– Preheat oven to 350°.

2– Sift cake mix into a large bowl, making a well in the center.

3– In a separate bowl, mix together egg subsititute, milk and oil, then add to the well in the cake mix.

4– Stir until well blended, then mix in chocolate chips, if desired.

5– Drop by teaspoonful on lightly sprayed cookie sheets.

6– Bake for 8–10 minutes at 350°.

343

Serving size:
1 cookie, with chocolate chips

Per Serving:
Calories: 58
Grams of carbohydrate: 10
Grams of protein: .8
Grams of fat: 1.7
¼Fa

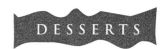

Cardiac Carrot Cake

344

Vegetable oil spray

4 cups carrots, grated (spooned, not packed, into cup)

2 cups sugar

8-ounce can crushed pineapple

1 cup prune butter
(see recipe on page 352)
or prune baby food

4 egg whites

2 teaspoons vanilla

2 cups flour

2 teaspoons baking soda

2 teaspoons cinnamon

½ teaspoon salt

¾ cup shredded coconut

Serving size:
1 piece without frosting

Per Serving:
Calories: 309
Grams of carbohydrate: 70
Grams of protein: 2
Grams of fat: 2
½S, ½V, ½Fr, ¼Fa (sugar)

This is a very good recipe plain, dusted with powdered sugar or frosted. For a low fat cream cheese frosting, combine in a mixing bowl: 12 ounces of low fat cream cheese, ½ cup confectioners sugar and 1½ teaspoons pure vanilla extract. Beat with an electric mixer until smooth and creamy.

Serves 12

1– Preheat oven to 375° and coat a 9" x 13" pan with vegetable spray.

2– In a large mixing bowl place carrots, sugar, pineapple, prune butter, egg whites and vanilla. Stir to blend.

3– Add remaining ingredients except coconut, mix thoroughly and then add coconut and stir just to mix.

4– Spread batter into pan and bake about 45 minutes or until a toothpick comes out clean.

5– Cool and cut into twelve equal pieces.

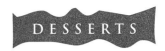
DESSERTS

Chocolate Hazelnut Meringues

¼ cup toasted,
  chopped hazelnuts

Parchment paper

3 egg whites,
  at room temperature

⅛ teaspoon cream of tartar

½ teaspoon vanilla extract

⅔ cup granulated sugar

¼ cup semisweet chocolate
  morsels, coarsely chopped

Serving size:
1 meringue

Per Serving:
Calories: 16
Grams of carbohydrates: 2.68
Grams of protein: 2.7
Grams of fat: .6
¼P

The flavor of the roasted hazelnuts with the chocolate is tantalizing. You can substitute other nuts, but the hazelnut is the ultimate for this recipe.

Yield: 50-60

1— Toast the hazelnuts on a cookie sheet in a preheated, 350° oven for 8 minutes.

2— Lower the oven temperature to 300° for baking the meringues.

3— Line baking sheets with parchment paper and set aside.

4— In a medium-large bowl, combine the egg whites with the cream of tartar and the vanilla. Beat at medium-high speed until soft peaks form.

5— Add the sugar slowly to the egg mixture, one tablespoon at a time, while beating. Beat until all of the sugar is incorporated and the mixture is stiff and glossy.

6— Using a large rubber spatula, fold in the chocolate morsels and the nuts.

7— Drop slightly rounded tablespoons onto parchment-lined baking sheets, allowing at least 1" between spoonfuls.

8— Bake for 30 minutes at 300°. Leaving the meringues in the oven, turn the oven off and allow cookies to sit in oven for at least 1 hour, until they are completely dry and crisp. Remove from oven and transfer to wire cooling racks.

345

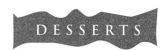

Chocolate Soufflé Tart

Decadent, delicious and definitely worth one fat serving. Beautiful served with raspberry fruit coulis and 3 whole fresh raspberries and mint leaves.

346

Serves 10

Vegetable oil spray

¼ cup toasted almonds (1 ounce)

Parchment paper

3 tablespoons all-purpose flour

3 ounces bittersweet or semisweet chocolate, chopped fine

½ cup unsweetened Dutch process cocoa

1 cup granulated sugar

½ cup boiling water

2 egg yolks

1 tablespoon brandy or Kahlúa

4 egg whites, at room temperature

¼ scant teaspoon cream of tartar

2–3 teaspoons confectioners sugar

Serving size:

1 piece

Per Serving:

Calories: 192
Grams of carbohydrates: 30.2
Grams of protein: 3.3
Grams of fat: 6.4
1Fa (sugar)

1– Toast almonds on an ungreased cookie sheet for 8 minutes at 350°. Then position oven rack in the lower third of oven and preheat to 375°.

2– Place a round of parchment paper in the bottom of a round, 8" springform pan, and spray the sides with vegetable oil.

3– In a food processor, grind the almonds with the flour until the texture is very fine. Set aside.

4– Combine the chopped chocolate, cocoa and ¾ cup of the granulated sugar in a large bowl. Pour in the boiling water and whisk until smooth and chocolate is completely melted.

5– Whisk in egg yolks and brandy or Kahlúa, then set aside.

6– Combine egg whites and cream of tartar in a medium bowl and beat at medium speed until soft peaks form. Gradually add the remaining sugar and beat on high speed until stiff but not dry.

7– Whisk the flour and almond mixture into the chocolate mixture. Fold approximately ¼ of the egg whites into this mix to lighten it, then fold in remaining egg whites.

8– Place batter in pan and level the top, if necessary. Bake 30–35 minutes, or until toothpick inserted in the center comes out with a few moist crumbs clinging to it.

9– Cool in the pan, atop a wire rack. Tart will sink in the middle like a soufflé.

10– Slide a knife between the tart and the pan, running it around the outside edge of the entire tart. Slide tart onto a platter and remove parchment paper.

11– Slice ten equal pieces and serve dusted with confectioners sugar.

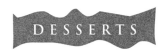

Fruit Coulis

1 pound fresh or frozen berries
(any kind)

1 tablespoon granulated sugar
(this is optional, and necessary
only to sweeten berries
if they are too tart)

2 tablespoons complementary
liqueur

Coulis is a sauce made from puréed fruits or vegetables. It can be used to coat the bottom of a plate, for added color and flavor, or drizzled over the top of a dish. This is a delicious, colorful, nonfat and simple choice instead of whipping cream.

Yield: 2 cups

1— If using frozen berries, thaw to room temperature, then pour off excess liquid. If using fresh berries, simply wash well and remove any stems.

2— Place berries in a food processor with a metal blade and purée.

347

3— Once fruit is puréed, pass it through a fine mesh sieve or a ricer to eliminate any seeds.

4— Sweeten the coulis with sugar if it is too tart, then stir in the liqueur.

Serving size:
2 tablespoons

Per Serving:
Calories: 18
Grams of carbohydrate: 4.5
Grams of protein: Trace
Grams of fat: Trace
¼Fr

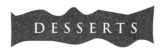

DESSERTS

Fudgy Cocoa Sauce

1 cup water

¾ cup granulated sugar

1 cup Dutch process cocoa powder

1 teaspoon pure vanilla extract

348

Substitute this sauce for the melted semisweet chocolate in your favorite fattening chocolate recipes. The higher quality cocoa you use, the better your sauce will be. Always use Dutch process cocoa.

Yield: 1 ½ cups

1– Combine the water and sugar in a small saucepan over medium heat and stir until sugar is dissolved.

2– Increase the heat and bring liquid to a boil for 1 full minute, to form a sugar syrup.

3– Remove from heat and whisk the cocoa powder into the mixture.

4– Return saucepan to medium heat and whisk until smooth and thick, about 3–5 minutes.

5– Remove from heat and mix in vanilla extract.

6– Let sauce cool completely. It will thicken slightly as it cools. Store the sauce in a tightly covered container in the refrigerator until ready to use.

Serving size:

2 tablespoons

Per Serving:

Calories: 42

Grams of carbohydrate: 8.3

Grams of protein: 7

Grams of fat: 7

No measurable food servings

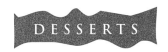

DESSERTS

Fuji Applesauce

24 Fuji apples, peeled, cored and
    quartered

2 pieces of fresh ginger

2 cups water

Other interesting ingredients:

Cinnamon and nutmeg to taste

Lemon zest

Fuji applesauce is a great side dish for a pork roast. It is also a wonderful, light dessert. I like to layer it in a pretty glass with crushed graham crackers and top it with some nonfat vanilla yogurt.

Serves 12

1– Place apples and ginger in a large pot and add water. Let simmer until soft. Every 15 minutes, mash apples with a potato masher.

2– Fujis take a long time to cook, maybe 1 hour. The applesauce is best if served warm.

349

Serving size:
1 cup

Per Serving:
Calories: 80
Grams of carbohydrate: 20
Grams of protein: 0
Grams of fat: Trace
2Fr

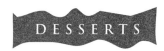

Kiwi Sorbet

2 cups water

½ cup sugar

6 kiwi fruit, peeled
and sliced

Water

Serves Eight

Serving size: ½ cup

Per Serving:
Calories: 64
Grams of carbohydrate: 16
Grams of protein: 0
Grams of fat: Trace
½Fr (sugar)

Most any berry could be substituted for the kiwi, like raspberry or blueberry.

1– In a saucepan over high heat, combine water and sugar. Stir until sugar dissolves.

2– Place kiwis and sugar water in blender or processor and puree.

3– Add enough water to make the whole mixture equal 4 cups.

4– Put in a Donvier ice cream maker and follow directions that come with the maker.

5– If you don't have a Donvier, freeze the mixture, then let thaw enough to put in a food processor and pulse until thick and creamy, then refreeze for future use or serve.

350

Lite Cream

2 cups nonfat ricotta cheese

6 tablespoons nonfat
vanilla yogurt

Pinch of salt

Serves 18

Use this as you would a crème fraîche or heavy cream.

1– Combine ingredients in a blender until smooth.

2– Store in refrigerator overnight for best results.

Serving size: 2 tablespoons

Per Serving:
Calories: 2.4   Grams of carbohydrate: 2
Grams of protein: 3.5   Grams of fat: Trace
¼D

Oatmeal Cookies

Vegetable oil spray

½ cup granulated sugar

½ cup dark brown sugar, packed

¼ cup butter, softened to room temperature

6 ounces prune butter (*see recipe on page 352*) or prune baby food, or 1 ripe banana

½ cup egg substitute

2 teaspoons vanilla

1 cup all-purpose flour

½ cup whole wheat flour

1½ teaspoons cinnamon

¼ teaspoon salt

1 teaspoon baking soda

2 cups oats, old-fashioned rolled

1 cup crispy rice cereal

¼ cup walnuts, chopped

½ cup raisins or dried cranberries

Serving size:

1 cookie

Per Serving:

Calories: 54

Grams of carbohydrate: 8

Grams of protein: 1

Grams of fat: 1.5

1S, ¼Fr, ¼Fa

This is a healthy treat for your kids' lunch boxes or for the times you have a craving for something sweet.

Yield: 5 dozen

1— Preheat oven to 350° and spray cookie sheets with vegetable oil spray.

2— Place sugars, butter and prune butter in a large bowl and cream together until blended. Add egg substitute and vanilla and beat well.

3— Mix together flours, cinammon, salt and soda in a separate bowl, then gradually blend into creamed mixture.

4— Stir in oats, crispy rice cereal, walnuts and raisins until blended.

5— Using a tablespoon, scoop up dough and drop on the prepared baking sheets, leaving about 2 inches between cookies.

6— Lightly press cookie with a fork to ¼" thickness. Bake for about 12–14 minutes.

351

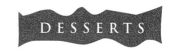

Prune Butter

⅓ cup pitted prunes

2 teaspoons corn syrup,
  light colored

2 tablespoons water

Prune butter can be substituted for half the fat in most cake recipes that are not white in color, like carrot cake or chocolate cake.

Yield: ½ cup

1– Combine all ingredients in a food processor and process until smooth.

352

Serving size:

½ cup

Per Serving:
Calories: 156
Grams of carbohydrate: 39
Grams of protein: Trace
Grams of fat: Trace
1Fr

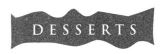

Whipped Cream

¼ cup cold water

¼ cup instant nonfat
  dry milk

Sugar and vanilla

There are some low fat whipped creams at the grocery store that are quite good. But if you feel like experimenting, try this recipe as a good substitute for whipped cream.

Serves 6-8

1— In a small bowl, whisk cold water and instant nonfat dry milk.

2— Chill in freezer for 40–50 minutes or until frozen, but not hard.

3— Beat the frozen mixture with an electric mixer at high speed for 5–7 minutes or until it whips into soft peaks.

4— Add a little sugar and vanilla for flavor.

353

Serving size:

3 tablespoons

Per Serving:
Calories: 15
Grams of carbohydrate: 3
Grams of protein: 1.6
Grams of fat: Trace
¼D

Drinks ·

Drinks should not be sought out only when you are thirsty.
They are a good alternative for a snack, and some hearty drinks can
even serve as a light meal.

When it's 4:00 P.M. and you've hit a low sugar point, throw some fresh berries,
nonfat milk and ice into a blender. This not only gives you a tasty milk shake
(with just a trace of fat), it also provides one of your daily servings of fruit
and dairy from the Food Pyramid.

In this recipe section, we give you several low fat, high taste choices.
They can be enjoyed any time of year and are great alternatives to alcoholic
beverages at parties and get-togethers.

354

Drinks

Banana Peanut Butter Shake
Blackberry Winter
Cranberry Orange Soda
Frozen Hot Chocolate
Piña Colada
Raspberry Banana Smoothie
Strawberry Banana Smoothie
Strawberry Orange Smoothie

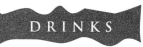

Banana Peanut Butter Shake

1 cup frozen nonfat vanilla yogurt

1 cup skim milk

1 medium frozen banana
  cut into 8 pieces

1 teaspoon peanut butter

5 cubes of ice

You can change the fruit in this shake to whatever is in season, but you might want to leave out the peanut butter. Without it, you'll have a fat-free shake.

Serves Two

Serving size: 8 ounces

Per Serving:

Calories: 185   Grams of carbohydrate: 30.5
Grams of protein: 12.5   Grams of fat: 1.25
1Fr, 1D, ¼Fa

1– Place all ingredients in blender. Cover and blend for 20–30 seconds.

356

Blackberry Winter

2 Blackcurrant tea bags

2 cups boiling water

½ cup apple-raspberry juice

1 lime, cut into slices

This tea offers a calming element to a busy day, a soothing end to a long evening, a gratifying moment of pleasure that should not be denied.

Serves Three

Serving size: ¾ cup

Per Serving:

Calories: 10
Grams of carbohydrate: 2.5
Grams of protein: 0   Grams of fat: 0
No measurable food servings

1– Place 2 tea bags and 2 cups boiling water in preheated tea pot. Let it steep for 2 minutes then remove tea bags.

2– Microwave juice for 30 seconds, then add to tea pot.

3– Serve in 3 teacups, and garnish each with a lime slice.

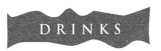

DRINKS

Cranberry Orange Soda

48 ounces Cranberry Juice
  Cocktail

1½ quarts Club Soda

2 oranges

Ice

Serves 24

1— Fill a large pitcher with ice.

2— Pour cranberry juice and club soda into the pitcher.

3— Cut the oranges into slices and cut each slice in half.
Add slices to the pitcher.

Serving size: 6 ounces

Per Serving:
Calories: 36   Grams of carbohydrate: 9
Grams of protein: 0   Grams of fat: 0
¼Fr

357

Frozen Hot Chocolate

½ cup unsweetened Dutch process
  cocoa

¾ cup sugar

2¾ cups nonfat milk

Serves Four

1— In a small saucepan, combine cocoa and sugar, stirring
in just enough of the milk to form a smooth paste.

2— Slowly stir in all but 2 tablespoons of the remaining milk.

3— Stir over low heat until the mixture is warm and the
sugar is dissolved.

4— Pour into a shallow pan and cover well. Freeze for at
least six hours or overnight.

5— Break frozen mixture into chunks with a fork or knife
and place chunks in a food processor with a metal blade.

6— Process with remaining 2 tablespoons of milk until no
lumps appear and mixture is thick and light in color.
Serve in frosted goblets.

Serving size: 6 ounces

Per Serving:
Calories: 144
Grams of carbohydrates: 29.6
Grams of protein: 4.6
Grams of fat: 2.3
½D, ½Fa (sugar)

DRINKS

Piña Colada

1 12-ounce can frozen pineapple juice

2 bananas, peeled, frozen and cut into chunks

4 teaspoons coconut milk

2 dozen ice cubes

Sometimes coconut milk is difficult to find. Williams-Sonoma carries a Taste of Thai "lite" coconut milk. This product is also good for other Thai cooking, as most other coconut milks are very high in fat.

Serves Four

1— Prepare the pineapple juice according to the instructions on the can.

2— Pour half of the prepared pineapple juice into a blender, then add the bananas, coconut milk and ice cubes and blend until smooth. Reserve the remaining pineapple juice for another batch of Piña Coladas!

Serving size: 1 cup

Per Serving:
Calories: 114
Grams of carbohydrate: 26
Grams of protein: 0   Grams of fat: 1
2Fr

358

Raspberry Banana Smoothie

½ cup orange juice

⅓ cup unsweetened frozen raspberries

½ medium banana, cut in 4 pieces

The next three smoothies are quick and tasty.

Serves One

1— Place all three ingredients in blender and blend for 15–20 seconds. What could be easier?

Serving size: 1 cup

Per Serving:
Calories: 100   Grams of carbohydrate: 25
Grams of protein: 0   Grams of fat: Trace
2½Fr

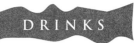
DRINKS

Strawberry Banana Smoothie

½ cup low fat buttermilk

⅓ cup frozen unsweetened strawberries

¼ cup skim milk

¼ medium banana, cut into pieces

2 teaspoons all-fruit marmalade (*optional*)

Serves One

1– Place all ingredients in blender and blend for 20–30 seconds.

Serving size: 10 ounces

Per Serving:
Calories: 134   Grams of carbohydrate: 25
Grams of protein: 6   Grams of fat: Trace
1Fr, ¾D

359

Strawberry Orange Smoothie

Serves One

½ cup orange juice

⅓ cup frozen unsweetened berries

½ cup nonfat vanilla yogurt

1– Put first two ingredients in blender and liquefy.

2– Add yogurt and blend about 5 seconds more.

Serving size: 10 ounces

Per Serving:
Calories: 120   Grams of carbohydrate: 26
Grams of protein: 4   Grams of fat: 0
1½Fr, ½D

Table of Equivalents

Dash	=	less than ⅛ teaspoon
3 teaspoons	=	1 tablespoon (½ fluid ounce)
2 tablespoons	=	⅛ cup (1 fluid ounce)
4 tablespoons	=	¼ cup (2 fluid ounces)
16 ounces	=	1 pound
8 tablespoons	=	½ cup (4 fluid ounces)
10⅔ tablespoons	=	⅔ cup (5⅓ fluid ounces)
12 tablespoons	=	¾ cup (6 fluid ounces)
14 tablespoons	=	⅞ cup (7 fluid ounces)
16 tablespoons	=	1 cup
1 cup	=	8 fluid ounces
2 cups	=	1 pint
2 pints	=	1 quart
4 quarts	=	1 gallon
1 gram	=	.035 ounces
1 ounce	=	28.35 grams
5⅓ tablespoons	=	⅓ cup (2⅔ fluid ounces)
1 coffee cup	=	Usually 6 ounces

360

Charts

Recommended Food Servings for Weight Loss
(based on weight and activity level)

Recommended Food Servings for Weight Maintenance
(based on weight and activity level)

Grocery List

Resting Heart Rate

Target Heart Rate Zone

Refined Sugar Recommendations

Recommended Food Servings for Weight Loss®*
(based on weight and activity level)

Little or No Activity

	100–120	120–140	140–160	160–180	180–200
Fat	1–2	2	2	2–3	3
Dairy	2	2	2	2	2–3
Protein	3	3–4	4–5	5–6	5–6
Vegetable	4	4–5	5	5	5–6
Fruit	3	3	3–4	4	4
Grain/Starch	5–7	7–9	9–10	10–12	12

Moderate Activity

	100–120	120–140	140–160	160–180	180–200
Fat	1–2	2	2	2–3	3
Dairy	2	2	2	2	2–3
Protein	3	3–4	4–5	5–6	5–6
Vegetable	4	4–5	5	5	5–6
Fruit	3	3	3–4	4	4
Grain/Starch	5–7	7–9	9–10	10–12	12

Vigorous Activity

	100–120	120–140	140–160	160–180	180–200
Fat	2	2	2–3	3	3
Dairy	2	2	2–3	3	3
Protein	4	4–6	6	6–8	6–8
Vegetable	4–5	5–6	6	6	6
Fruit	3–4	4	4	4	4–5
Grain/Starch	7–9	9–10	10–11	11–12	12–14

362

These numbers differ from those given by the U.S. Department of Agriculture. The USDA's numbers are lower and do not account for physical activity. The numbers above are estimates and may change based on your individual metabolism, lifestyle, etc.

FAT CHANCE

Recommended Food Servings for Weight Maintenance®*
(based on weight and activity level)

Little or No Activity

	100–120	120–140	140–160	160–180	180–200
Fat	2	2	2–3	3	3
Dairy	2	2	2–3	3	3
Protein	3–4	4–6	6	6–8	6–8
Vegetable	4–5	5–6	6	6	6
Fruit	3	4	4	4	4–5
Grain/Starch	7–9	9–10	10–11	11–12	12–14

Moderate Activity

	100–120	120–140	140–160	160–180	180–200
Fat	2	2–3	3	3	3–4
Dairy	2	2–3	3	3	3–4
Protein	4–6	6	6–8	6–8	8
Vegetable	5–6	6	6	6	6
Fruit	4	4	4	4–5	5
Grain/Starch	9–10	10–11	11–12	12–14	14–15

Vigorous Activity

	100–120	120–140	140–160	160–180	180–200
Fat	2–3	3	3	3–4	4
Dairy	2–3	3	3	3–4	4
Protein	6	6–8	8	8	8–10
Vegetable	6	6	6	6	6–7
Fruit	4	4	4–5	5	5
Grain/Starch	11–12	12–13	13–14	14–15	15–16

363

These numbers differ from those given by the U.S. Department of Agriculture. The USDA's numbers are lower and do not account for physical activity. The numbers above are estimates and may change based on your individual metabolism, lifestyle, etc.

Grocery List

Dairy

Butter—lite

Canadian Bacon

Cottage cheese—nonfat

Cream cheese—nonfat

Egg substitute

Eggs

Cheese—nonfat Cheddar,
    Mozzarella & Ricotta

Hot Dogs—nonfat

Milk—nonfat

Parmesan cheese—
    grated/whole

Pasta—fresh

Pudding/Gelatin—nonfat

Sour cream—nonfat

Tortillas—low fat

Drinks

Beer

Club soda/tonic

Gatorade

Soda—Rootbeer/7-Up/Orange

Paper Goods

Foil

Napkins—regular

Paper towels

Plastic bags (sandwich/
    quart/gal/jumbo)

Plastic/styrofoam cups

Plastic wrap

Plates

Tissue

Toilet paper

Trash bags

Cleaning Supplies

Bathroom cleaner

Bleach

Cleanser

Dish soap

Dishwasher soap

Furniture polish

Laundry detergent

Baby

Baby shampoo

Diapers

Fever reducer

Formula

Ointment

Wipes

Deli

Cheese—lite

Ham—lite

Roast Beef—lite

Turkey—lite

Basics

Beans—
    kidney/refried/garbanzo

Cereal—low fat

Chicken/beef/vegetable broth—
    nonfat

Coffee—decaf/regular

Cornstarch

Dressings—nonfat

Jam—all fruit

Ketchup

Mayonnaise—lite

Oil—olive/canola

Peanut butter—old-fashioned

Rice—white/brown/wild/mixed

Salt/pepper/garlic powder

Seasoning packets

Soup—reduced fat

Soy sauce—lite

Tea—regular/decaf

Tuna—packed in water

Basics— Baking

Baking mixes

Baking powder

Baking soda

Dutch process cocoa

Flour

Oats

Sugar—granulated/brown/
    powdered

Vanilla

Frozen Foods

Frozen yogurt—nonfat

Ice cream—Lite

Juice

Lemonade

Petite peas

Non-Grocery

Aspirin

Bar Soap

Batteries

Deodorant

Dog/cat food

Hair spray

Lotion

Sanitary napkins

Shampoo/Conditioner

Shaving cream

Toothpaste

364

Snacks

Bagel Crisp—fat-free

Butterscotch

Caramel popcorn—nonfat

Chips—low fat

Chocolate sauce

Cookies—fat-free

Lemon drops

Licorice—red

Oriental snack mix

Popcorn

Pretzels—fat-free

Fruit

Apples

Bananas

Berries

Cantaloupe

Grapefruit

Grapes

Lemons/limes

Melons

Oranges

Peaches

Pears

Pineapple

Plums

Strawberries

Tangerines

Watermelon

Vegetables

Artichokes

Asparagus

Avocado

Beans

Broccoli

Brussels sprouts

Cabbage—curly

Carrots/celery

Cauliflower

Chinese noodles—fresh

Corn

Cucumbers

Garlic/shallots

Lettuce—romaine/head/butter
    red leaf/green leaf

Mushrooms—whole/sliced

Onions—yellow/red/green

Parsley/cilantro/basil

Peppers—red/yellow/green

Pine nuts

Potatoes—russet/new/sweet

Spinach

Swiss chard

Tomatoes

Zucchini, light green

Bread

Bagels—nonfat

Buns—hamburger/hot dog

Crumpets

Cubes/crumbs

French baguettes

Sandwich—brown

Sourdough—rolls/loaves

Meat & Fish

Beef—steaks/roast/loin

Chicken—whole/breast/fillets

Fish

Hamburger—lean

Lamb—rack/roast/chops

Pork—loin/chops

Turkey—whole/breast/fillets

Pasta—Dried

Butterfly

Lasagne

Linguine

Penne

Shells

Spaghetti

Dry Cleaners

Take—Pickup

Extras

_____

_____

_____

_____

_____

_____

_____

_____

_____

_____

_____

_____

_____

_____

_____

_____

365

Resting Heart Rate

A good estimate of your resting heart rate can be obtained if you count your pulse before getting out of bed in the morning. Lay back and relax, and find your pulse (at your wrist or neck). Count the number of beats for one full minute. Do this for three days and take the average of the days to get your resting heart rate.

CALCULATING YOUR RESTING RATE

Resting Heart Rate	Day 1	Day 2	Day 3
	_____	_____	_____
Total of all days	_____ ÷ 3 = _____ Average Resting Heart Rate		

Target Heart Rate Zone

While doing aerobic exercise, your heart rate should remain in a zone that is safe and effective for your age and level of fitness. Your target heart rate zone represents this zone, which is actually a range between 65% and 80% of your maximum heart rate. Target heart rate zones are individual, and will vary from person to person. The chart below will determine your individual zone.

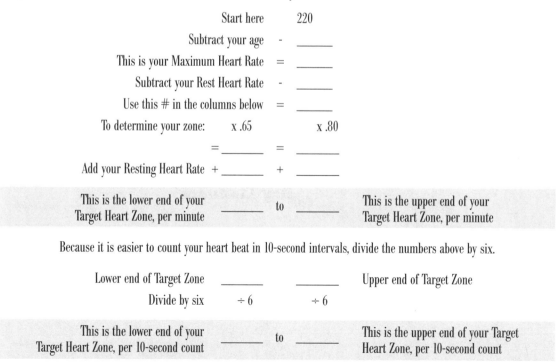

Start here	220		
Subtract your age	- _____		
This is your Maximum Heart Rate	= _____		
Subtract your Rest Heart Rate	- _____		
Use this # in the columns below	= _____		
To determine your zone:	x .65		x .80
	= _____		= _____
Add your Resting Heart Rate	+ _____		+ _____

This is the lower end of your Target Heart Zone, per minute	_____ to _____	This is the upper end of your Target Heart Zone, per minute

Because it is easier to count your heart beat in 10-second intervals, divide the numbers above by six.

Lower end of Target Zone	_____	_____	Upper end of Target Zone
Divide by six	÷ 6	÷ 6	

This is the lower end of your Target Heart Zone, per 10-second count	_____ to _____	This is the upper end of your Target Heart Zone, per 10-second count

Target Heart Rate Zone

The shaded areas below designate the target training zones for exercising at an intensity that is moderate to hard, based on age.

Numbers are based on a 10-second count

Percentage of Maximum Heart Rate

Age	60%	65%	70%	75%	80%	85%
20	20	22	23	25	27	28
25	20	21	23	24	26	28
30	19	21	22	24	25	27
35	19	20	22	23	25	26
40	18	20	21	23	24	26
45	18	19	20	22	23	25
50	17	18	20	21	23	24
55	17	18	19	21	22	24
60	16	17	19	20	21	23
65	16	17	18	20	21	22
70	15	16	17	19	20	22
75	15	15	17	18	19	21

367

Refined Sugar Recommendations

The average American consumes more than 120 pounds of refined sugar per year—most of which comes from packaged foods. Although no measurable standards for total sugar intake have been set, research shows that an excess of refined sugar upsets the body's chemical balance and can increase your risk for cavities, diabetes and obesity. Therefore, we recommend you try to limit your total refined sugar intake to 10% of your daily calories. The table below reflects this moderate recommendation.

	Recommended Teaspoons per Day		
Weight	Little or No Exercise	Moderate Exercise	Vigorous Exercise
≤110	7	8	9
120	8	9	10
130	8	10	11
140	9	11	12
150	10	11	13
160	10	12	14
170	11	13	14
180	12	14	15
190	12	14	16
200	13	15	17

References

American College of Sports Medicine. 1990. *The Recommended Quantity and Quality of Exercise for Developing and Maintaining Cardiorespiratory and Muscular Fitness in Healthy Adults.*

American College of Sports Medicine. 1992. *Guidelines for Exercise Testing and Prescription.* Philadelphia: Lea and Febiger Publishing.

Anderson, Ross E. 1991. Weights for Over Weights. *Fitness Management.* 6/91, 44–45.

Baggett, Nancy and Glick, Ruth. 1994. *100% Pleasure.* Pennsylvania: Rodale Books.

Bailey, Covert. 1994. *Smart Exercise.* New York: Houghton Mifflin Company.

Bennett, William and Gurin, Joel. 1982. *The Dieter's Dilemma: Eating Less and Weighing More.* New York: Basic Books.

Blackburn, G.L., Wilson, G.T., Kanders, B.S., Stein, L.J., Lavin, P.T., Adler, J., and Brownell, K.D. 1989. Weight Cycling: The Experience of Human Dieters. *American Journal of Clinical Nutrition.* 49: 1105–1109.

Browne, Mona Boyd, contrib. and comp. 1993. *Label Facts for Healthful Living.* National Food Processors Association. Dayton: The Mazer Corporation.

Brownell, K.D. 1990. Dieting Readiness. *The Weight Control Digest.* 1(1): 1, 5–9.

Brownell, K.D., Marlatt, G.A., Lichtenstein, E., and Wilson, G.T. 1986. Understanding and Preventing Relapse. *American Psychologist.* 41(7): 765–782.

Cash, T.F. 1992. Body Images and Body Weight: What Is There to Gain or Lose? *The Weight Control Digest.* 2(4): 169, 172–176.

Claiborne, Craig. 1990. *The New York Times Cook Book.* New York: Harper & Row.

Consumer Reports. 1993. Losing Weight: What Works, What Doesn't. June, 1993. 347–359.

Cooper, Kenneth H., and Cooper, Mildred. 1988. *The New Aerobics for Women.* New York: Bantam Books.

Cooper, Robert K. 1989. *Health and Fitness Excellence: The Scientific Action Plan.* Boston: Houghton Mifflin Company.

Daley, Rosie. 1994. *In the Kitchen with Rosie.* New York: Alfred A. Knopf, Inc.

Donovan, Mary Deirdre, ed. 1993. Culinary Institute of America. *Techniques of Healthy Cooking.* New York: Van Nostrand Reinhold.

Doyle, Bob, ed. 1995. *Sunset Recipe Annual 1996.* Menlo Park: Sunset Publishing Corporation.

Ets-Hokin, Judith. 1975. *The San Francisco Dinner Party Cookbook.* Boston: Houghton Mifflin Company.

Evans, William, and Rosenberg, Irwin H. 1992. *Biomarkers*. New York: Fireside.

Famularo, Joseph J., and Imperiale, Louise. 1983. *The Joy of Pasta*. New York: Barron's Educational Series, Inc.

Farmer, Fannie Merritt. 1965. *The Fannie Farmer Cookbook*. Boston: Little, Brown and Company.

Ferguson, K.J., Brink, P.J., Wood, M., and Koop, P.M. 1992. Characteristics of Successful Dieters as Measured by Guided Interview Responses and Restraint Scale Scores. *Journal of the American Dietetic Association*. 92(9): 1119–1121.

Fitzgibbon, M.L., and Kirschenbaum, D.S. 1992. Who Succeeds in Losing Weight? In J.D. Fisher, J. Chinsky, Y. Klan and A. Nadler, eds. *Initiating Self-Changes: Social Psychological and Clinical Perspectives*. 153–175. New York: Springer-Verlag.

Fitzpatrick, Nancy J., ed. 1993. *Cooking Light Cookbook*. Birmingham: Oxmoor House, Inc.

Flatt, J.P. 1987. Dietary Fat, Carbohydrate Balance and Weight Maintenance: Effects of Exercise. *American Journal of Clinical Nutrition*. 45.

Food and Nutritional Board, National Research Council, National Academy of Sciences. 1980. *Recommended Dietary Allowances*. Washington, D.C.

Foreyt, J.P., and Goodrick, G.K. 1991. Choosing the Right Weight Management Program. *The Weight Control Digest*. 1(6): 81, 84–90.

Frederick, Sue. 1992. *The Delicious! Collection: Simple Recipes for Healthy Living*. Boulder: New Hope Communications, Inc.

Galloway, Jeff. 1984. *Galloway's Book on Running*. Bolinas: Shelter Publications, Inc.

Gavin, J. 1992. *The Exercise Habit*. Champaign: Leisure Press.

Gershoff, Stanley, ed. 1990. *The Tufts University Guide to Total Nutrition*. New York: Harper & Row.

Goldstein, Joyce Esersky. 1978. *Feedback*. New York: Richard Marek Publishers.

Goldstein, Joyce. 1989. *The Mediterranean Kitchen*. New York: William Morrow and Company, Inc.

Goldstein, Joyce. 1992. *Back to Square One*. New York: William Morrow and Company, Inc.

Gray, D.S., et al. 1988. Effects of Repeated Weight Loss and Regain on Body Composition in Obese Rats. *American Journal of Clinical Nutrition*. 47.

Grilo, C.M., and Brownell, K.D. 1993. Relapse: Why, How and What to Do about It. *The Weight Control Digest*. 3(1): 217, 220–224.

Grilo, C.M., Shiffman, S., and Wing, R.R. 1989. Relapse Crises and Coping Among Dieters. *Journal of Consulting and Clinical Psychology*. 57(4): 488–495.

Grilo, C.M., Wilfley, D.E., and Brownell, K.D. 1992. Physical Activity and Weight Control: Why Is the Link So Strong? *The Weight Control Digest*. 2(3): 153, 157–160.

Junior League of Oakland-East Bay, The. 1985. *California Fresh*. Oakland: The Junior League of Oakland-East Bay, Inc.

Junior League of Sacramento, The. 1991. *Celebrate!* Sacramento: The Junior League of Sacramento, Inc.

369

Junior League of San Diego, The. 1988. *Delicious Decisions*. San Diego: The Junior League of San Diego, Inc.

Junior League of San Francisco, The. 1979. *San Francisco á la Carte*. San Francisco: The Junior League of San Francisco, Inc.

Katzen, Mollie. 1992. *Moosewood Cookbook*. Berkeley: Ten Speed Press.

Kerr, Graham. 1991. *Smart Cooking*. New York: Doubleday.

Kerr, Graham. 1992. *Graham Kerr's Minimax Cookbook*. New York: Doubleday.

Kolpas, Norman, and Williams, Chuck, Ed. 1993. *Williams-Sonoma Kitchen Library: Soups*. New York: Time Life Books.

Marshall, Lydie. 1995. *Chez Nous*. New York: HarperCollins.

McNutt, Heidi. 1992. *New Dieter's Cook Book*. Des Moines: Better Homes and Gardens Books.

Moskowitz, H.R., ed. 1987. Fats and Food Texture: Sensory and Hedonic Evaluations. *Food Texture*. New York: Marcel Dekker.

O'Connor, Jill. 1993. *Sweet Nothings*. San Francisco: Chronicle Books.

Ornish, Dean. 1990. *Dr. Dean Ornish's Program for Reversing Heart Disease*. New York: Random House.

Ornish, Dean. 1993. *Eat More, Weigh Less*. New York: HarperCollins.

Pennington, Jean A.T. 1989. *Bowes & Church's Food Values of Portions Commonly Used*. Philadelphia: J.B. Lippincott Company.

Pépin, Jacques. 1992. *Good Life Cooking: Light Classics from Today's Gourmet*. San Francisco: KQED, Inc.

Perri, M.G. 1992. Weight Maintenance Strategies: The Process and Practice. *Weight Control Digest*. 2(6): 201, 204–207.

Polivy, J., and Herman, C.P. 1983. *Breaking the Diet Habit*. New York: Basic Books.

Prewitt, T.E., Schmeisser, D., Bowen, P.E., Aye, P., Dolecek, T.E., Langenberg, P., Cole, T., and Brace, L. 1991. Changes In Body Weight, Body Composition, and Energy Intake in Women Fed High and Low Fat Diets. *American Journal of Clinical Nutrition*. 54: 304–310.

Rippe, J.M., et al. 1988. Walking for Health and Fitness. *Journal of the American Medical Association*. 259.

Rombauer, Irma S., and Becker, Marion Rombauer. 1975. *The Joy of Cooking*. New York: Bobbs-Merrill Company, Inc.

Rosso, Julee, and Lukins, Sheila. 1982. *The Silver Palate Cookbook*. New York: Workman Publishing Company, Inc.

Rosso, Julee, and Lukins, Sheila. 1989. *The New Basics Cookbook*. New York: Workman Publishing Company, Inc.

Rosso, Julee. 1993. *Great Good Food*. New York: Crown Publishers, Inc.

Schneider, Sally. 1990. *The Art of Low Calorie Cooking*. New York: Stewart, Tabori & Chang, Inc.

370

Shepherd, R., and Stockley, L. 1985. Fat Consumption and Attitudes toward Food with a High Fat Content. *Human Nutrition: Applied Nutrition.* 39.

Shulman, Martha Rose. 1994. *Provençal Light.* New York: Bantam Books.

Slomon, Evelyne. 1984. *The Pizza Book.* New York: Times Books.

Smith, Linda Wasmer. 1995. Forever Young: Can a Meatless Diet Be Your Secret to Ageless Health? *Veggie Life.* 5/95: 39–41.

Somerville, Annie. 1993. *Fields of Greens.* New York: Bantam Books.

Szekely, Deborah, and Rancho La Puerta. 1990. *Vegetarian Spa Cuisine from Rancho La Puerta.* Escondido: Rancho La Puerta, Inc.

U.S. Department of Agriculture. 1975. *Nutritive Value of American Foods in Common Units.* Agriculture Handbook No. 456. Washington D.C.: GPO.

U.S. Department of Agriculture. 1989. *Composition of Foods.* Agriculture Handbook No. 8. Washington D.C.: GPO.

U.S. Department of Agriculture. 1995. *Report of the Dietary Guidelines Advisory Committee on the Dietary Guidelines for Americans.* Washington D.C.: GPO.

U.S. Department of Health and Human Services. 1988. *The Surgeon General's Report on Nutrition and Health.* DHHS (PHS) Publication No. 88–50210. Washington D.C.: GPO.

Wescott, W.L. 1990. *Strength Training Fitness: Physiological Principles and Training Technologies.* Dubuque: Wm. C. Brown Publishing.

Whitehouse, Frederick A. 1977. Motivation for Fitness. *Guide to Fitness after Fifty.* New York: Plenum.

Worthington, Diane Rossen. 1983. *The Cuisine of California.* New York: G.P. Putnam's Sons.

Additional References include, but are not limited to, the following:

American Health

American Heart Association

American Journal of Clinical Nutrition

Johns Hopkins Medical Letter

Journal of the American Dietetic Association

Mayo Clinic Health Letter

Medicine and Science in Sports and Exercise (ACSM Journal)

New England Journal of Medicine

Nutrition Action Healthletter

Penn State Sports Medicine Newsletter

Prevention Magazine

Runner's World Magazine

The Cooper Institute for Aerobics Research

The Edell Health Letter

The Weight Control Digest

Tufts University Diet and Nutrition Letter

U.S. Department of Health and Human Services

University of California at Berkeley Wellness Letter

Women's Sport and Fitness

371

Recipe Index

372

373

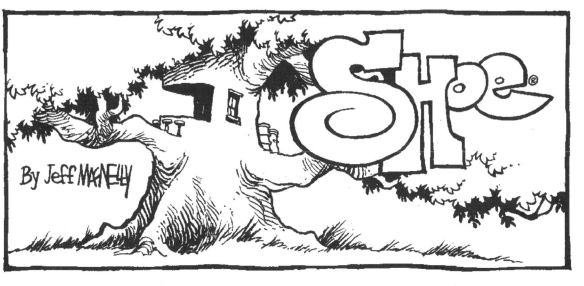

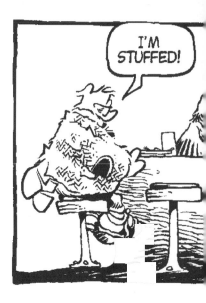

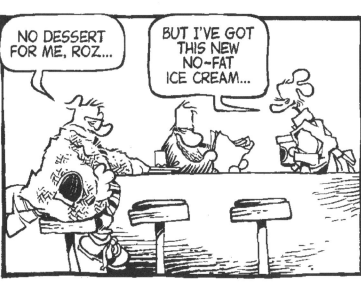

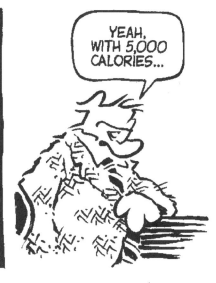

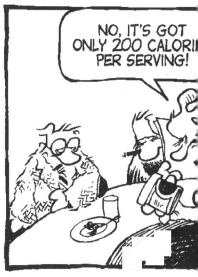

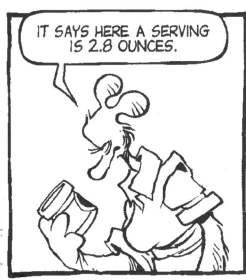

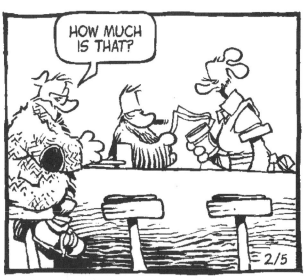

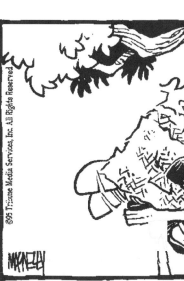